THE COMPLETE GUIDE TO
Everyday Risks
in
Pregnancy
&
Breastfeeding

✿ ✿ ✿ ✿ ✿

Answers To Your Questions
About Morning Sickness, Medications, Herbs, Diseases, Chemical Exposures & More

Dr. Gideon Koren, MD, FRCP(C)

FROM THE MOTHERISK PROGRAM AT THE HOSPITAL FOR SICK CHILDREN

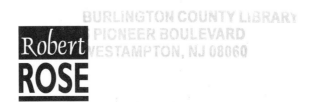

Robert
ROSE

The publisher acknowledges the financial support of the Government of Canada through the Book Publishing Industry Development Program.

The author would like to thank Susan Santiago, whose contribution to the writing and editing of this guide helped make the topics of teratogenicity and maternal-fetal toxicology understandable to all those who will read this book. He is also indebted to Dr. Michael Tan and Ms. Myla Moretti for their review and assistance.

The research presented in this book was supported by the Canadian Institute for Health Research; Lawson Foundation; Research Leadership for Better Pharmacotherapy During Pregnancy and Lactation; Ivey Chair in Molecular Toxicology (University of Western Ontario); The Hospital for Sick Children — Tel Aviv University Exchange Program; Jonathan's Alert; Duchesnay Inc; Novartis Inc; and Janssen Ortho Inc.

The nutritional, medical, and health information presented in this book is based on the research, training, and professional experience of the author, and is true and complete to the best of his knowledge. However, this book is intended only as an informative guide for those wishing to know more about health, nutrition, and medicine; it is not intended to replace or countermand the advice given by the reader's personal physician. Because each person and situation is unique, the author and the publisher urge the reader to check with a qualified health-care professional before using any procedure where there is a question as to its appropriateness. A physician should be consulted before beginning any exercise program. The author and the publisher are not responsible for any adverse effects or consequences resulting from the use of the information in this book. It is the responsibility of the reader to consult a physician or other qualified health-care professional regarding his or her personal care.

Library and Archives Canada Cataloguing in Publication

Koren, Gideon, 1947-
      The complete guide to everyday risks in pregnancy & breastfeeding : answers to your questions about medications, morning sickness, herbs, diseases, chemical exposures and more / Gideon Koren.

Based on the Motherisk Progam at Hospital for Sick Children, Toronto ON.
Includes bibliographical references and index.
ISBN 0-7788-0084-9

1. Prenatal care—Popular works. 2. Pregnancy—Popular works. 3. Breast feeding.
4. Pregnant women—Health and hygiene. I. Motherisk Program. II. Title.

RG525.K67 2004   618.2'4   C2004-902918-5

Edited by Bob Hilderley, Senior Editor, Health.
Copyedited by Fina Scroppo.
Design and page composition by PageWave Graphics Inc.

Published by Robert Rose Inc.
120 Eglinton Ave. E., Suite 800, Toronto, Ontario, Canada M4P 1E2
Tel: (416) 322-6552 Fax: (416) 322-6936.

Printed and bound in Canada.

1 2 3 4 5 6 7 8 9 CPL 12 11 10 09 08 07 06 05 04

Contents

The Ten Commandments for a Safe and Healthy Pregnancy

❶ Plan Your Pregnancy

Planning your pregnancy will help reduce the risk of potentially harmful exposures to teratogens (unsafe drugs, chemicals, and infections) once you are pregnant, and prevent conditions such as neural tube defects that can develop in the very earliest stages of fetal development. Also, if you have a chronic health condition, this is the time to talk to specialists about optimal therapy during pregnancy. If, however, your pregnancy is unplanned, don't worry. Nearly one-half of all pregnancies are not planned, and yet the vast majority of children born in North America are normal and healthy. Still, you'll want to get the facts on the Do's and Don'ts of drug and other exposures from the experts.

❷ Be Informed

This is where the experts come in. Though friends and family mean well, they may not be the best source of clinically sound advice. Nor should you believe everything you read on the internet. Your health-care provider and/or local teratogen information service should be your first call whenever you have a question about the risk or safety of drugs and other exposures in pregnancy.

❸ Take Folic Acid

You should start taking at least 0.4 mg of folic acid each day in the month or two before you conceive. Folic acid supplementation prevents neural tube defects and other possible malformations. Most prenatal vitamins have at least twice this recommended amount of folic acid, so start taking a prenatal vitamin while planning your pregnancy. If your pregnancy is unplanned, prenatal vitamin supplementation is still an important source of vitamins, iron, calcium, and other minerals.

❹ Do Not Self-Prescribe

You may be used to treating your coughs and colds, aches and pains with one or more of the thousand of products for sale at your local drug store, but now that you are pregnant (or planning a pregnancy), over-the-counter self-help ends. What is safe for you may not be safe for your unborn baby. Seek advice from your health-care provider or one of the local teratogen information centers listed in the "Resources" section of this book.

> **Teratogens**
>
> Teratogens are substances or environmental factors that can cause birth defects and other adverse fetal outcomes. In order for a drug, chemical, or infection to be considered a teratogen, there must be substantive evidence that being exposed to it causes birth defects.

⑤ Do Not Stop Medications for Chronic Conditions 'Cold Turkey'

Here again you'll want to get expert advice. Many medications do not pose a risk to the fetus. What's more, if you have relied on certain prescription medications to control conditions such as hypertension and depression, you may do more harm than good by suddenly going off your medication. Often you can continue your medication during pregnancy, but sometimes your doctor will want to prescribe another, safer medication. Also remember that many untreated conditions themselves pose a risk to the fetus. If you have a chronic medical condition and are planning a pregnancy, it is advisable to get that condition under control with the help of a medical specialist who is experienced with the management of pregnancy.

⑥ Do Not Drink Alcohol

Though we are learning more and more about the potentially devastating effects of alcohol drinking during pregnancy, we still do not know what level of alcohol consumption during pregnancy is safe. Once you plan to become pregnant or know that you are pregnant, stop drinking alcohol. If you find that quitting is a challenge, then speak to your health-care provider or teratogen counselor about where to go for help and support.

⑦ Be Smoke Free

When you smoke, your baby smokes. Maternal smoking has been shown to increase the risk of miscarriage, stillbirth, prematurity, and Sudden Infant Death Syndrome (SIDS). Cigarette smoke (either yours or your partner's) can compromise your health and the health of your unborn child. For many women, pregnancy is a powerful motivator for all sorts of healthy lifestyle changes. Planning a pregnancy? Then plan to quit smoking. Already pregnant? Then now is the time to make important changes for the sake of your unborn baby and yourself. Need help? Talk to your physician for more information on smoking cessation in pregnancy.

8 Know What You're Handling at Work

If your occupation involves exposure to chemicals, find out what chemicals are involved and seek advice as to their fetal safety. Here again, your local teratogen information service can help.

9 Be Cautious with Herbal Medicines

The key is to be guided by evidence-based information about the risk or safety of the medicines and products you use during pregnancy. In general, we have more information on the safety of older medications than on newer medications. When it comes to herbal medicines, there is little human safety data for safety or risk in pregnancy.

10 Proceed with Confidence!

There is plenty of excellent, evidence-based information to guide you throughout your pregnancy and while you breastfeed your child. Much of it is contained in the pages of this book. More importantly, though, your physician or other health-care providers are there to guide you. Ask questions, be positive, learn the facts. The list of known teratogens (medications, chemicals, and infections that have been proven to be unsafe to the unborn baby) is relatively short. The list of drugs that are not compatible with breastfeeding is even shorter. Stay informed and your chance of having a safe pregnancy and healthy baby are excellent.

RESOURCES

Teratogen Information Services

There are a number of teratogen information services in Europe, Israel, South America, and North America.

European Network Teratogen Information Services (ENTIS)

For local teratogen information services in Europe, Israel, and parts of South America, see the list of ENTIS members at www.entis-org.com.

Organization of Teratology Information Services (OTIS)

For local teratogen information services in most states and provinces in North America, contact OTIS Information at: (866) 626-OTIS or (866) 626-6847. Information about OTIS is also available on-line at www.otispregnancy.org/index.htm.

Motherisk

The Motherisk Program at The Hospital for Sick Children in Toronto, Canada is one of the largest teratogen research, counseling, and education centers in the world. Contact Motherisk on-line at www.motherisk.org or by telephone at (416) 813-6780.

Helpful Terms

There are a few basic scientific terms that you may want to know to help you understand the risk factors in pregnancy. You might want to bookmark this section and return to it when you encounter one of our more technical words.

Teratology
This is the medical science of abnormal development.

Toxicology
This is the science that deals with adverse effects of medications and chemicals on living systems, including plants, animals, and humans.

Organogenesis
This refers to the process of formation of the body's organs.

Congenital
This means "present at birth."

Congenital Malformation
This is the result of abnormal development of an organ, such as the heart or a limb. The medication thalidomide caused children to be born without parts of their limbs or without whole limbs. Brain development is also susceptible to congenital malformation. For example, the acne drug Accutane when taken by a pregnant woman may cause the exposed child to be developmentally delayed and to have a low IQ (intelligence quotient). Major malformations are defined as those that affect either the health or quality of life of the child. Often, major malformations can only be corrected through surgery.

Syndrome
This means the aggregate of signs and symptoms associated with a disease or disorder. Taken together, these signs and symptoms give a picture of the disease or disorder.

Evidence-Based Research
This refers to the systematic review, critical appraisal, and unbiased synthesis of clinical and experimental data and results.

Quick Guide to Selected Drugs and Chemicals Unsafe in Pregnancy

A number of common drugs and chemicals have been proven to cause malformations in the fetus when the mother has been exposed to them. This short list of known teratogens is derived from the comprehensive lists provided in succeeding chapters. Look ahead for more information and add your own notes to this list as you work through the book. Drugs marked with an asterisk * are not currently in clinical use.

DRUGS AND CHEMICALS	TERATOGENIC EFFECT
Alcohol *Notes:*	Fetal Alcohol Spectrum Disorder.
Alkylating Agents Anticancer drugs such as busulfan, chlorambucil, cyclophosphamide, mechlorethamine *Notes:*	Growth retardation, cleft palate, heart defects, and other anomalies.
Antimetabolic Agents Anticancer drugs such as aminopterin,* azauridine, cytarabine, 5-FU, 6-MP, methotrexate *Notes:*	Hydrocephalus and other developmental anomalies; skull, ear, eye, palate, and limb malformations.
Carbamazepine *Notes:*	Increased risk for neural tube defects.

DRUGS AND CHEMICALS	TERATOGENIC EFFECT
Carbon Monoxide *Notes:*	Cerebral atrophy, mental retardation, microcephaly, convulsions, spastic disorders, intrauterine or postnatal death.
Danazol and other Androgenic Drugs *Notes:*	Masculinization of female fetuses.
Diethylstilbestrol (DES)* *Notes:*	Vaginal carcinoma in female offspring and other genitourinary defects in female and male offspring.
Hypoglycemic Drugs *Notes:*	Hypoglycemia in the newborn.
Lead *Notes:*	Lower scores in developmental tests.
Lithium *Notes:*	Ebstein's anomaly of the heart.

DRUGS AND CHEMICALS	TERATOGENIC EFFECT
Methyl Mercury **Mercuric Sulfide** *Notes:*	Microcephaly, eye malformations, cerebral palsy, mental retardation, malocclusion of teeth.
Misoprostol *Notes:*	Moebius sequence (paralysis of cranial nerves).
Nonsteroidal Anti-inflammatory Drugs (NSAIDs) Such as aspirin, ibuprofen, naproxen *Notes:*	Possible gastroschisis. When used in third trimester, may prematurely close the fetal ductus arteriosus.
Paramethadione* *Notes:*	Facial and central nervous system defects.
PCBs (polychlorinated biphenyls) *Notes:*	Stillbirth. Children who survive do not meet milestones and show signs of central nervous system damage.
Penicillamine *Notes:*	Skin hyperelastosis.

DRUGS AND CHEMICALS	TERATOGENIC EFFECT
Phenytoin *Notes:*	Growth retardation and central nervous system damage.
Systemic Retinoids Such as isotretinoin (Accutane) and etretinate *Notes:*	Central nervous system damage, skull, face, heart, and other defects.
Tetracycline *Notes:*	Anomalies of teeth.
Thalidomide *Notes:*	Limb-shortening defects, internal organ defects.
Trimethadione* *Notes:*	Defects to face and central nervous system.
Valproic Acid *Notes:*	Neural tube defects.
Warfarin *Notes:*	Skeletal and central nervous system defects, Dandy-Walker syndrome.

Eight-Step Program for Planning a Safe and Healthy Pregnancy

Planning is a big part of a successful pregnancy. You'll want to think about everything from your emotional and financial readiness for raising a child to more immediate concerns about finding the right caregiver and support during and after pregnancy. All of those are important matters we shall leave to others. Since our unique expertise is the science of teratology, we will review the steps you can take to decrease the risk of teratogenic exposure, even before you are pregnant.

➊ Take Folic Acid to Prevent Neural Tube Defects

Why is folic acid so important before pregnancy? It's simple. By taking sufficient amounts of folic acid, you decrease dramatically the risk of spina bifida and other forms of neural tube defects. Neural tube defects are major congenital anomalies of the brain or spinal cord that occur when the brain or spine fails to close properly. This crucial event occurs very early in pregnancy — so early in fact, that many women run the risk of a neural tube defect even before they know they have conceived.

Folic acid is one of the B vitamins, found naturally in green leafy vegetables, nuts, and oranges. In North America, flour is fortified with folic acid and so it will appear in breads and pastas. By eating at least 400 micrograms of folic acid every day, the risk of neural tube defects decreases by 75%. But most women and men do not get that much through their daily diet. That is why women planning for pregnancy should take a supplement tablet containing folic acid every day. The best way to do this is to start taking a prenatal multiple vitamin pill that you intend to take later in pregnancy *before* you become pregnant, or even better — if you have unprotected sex. Ensure that your unborn child is protected.

▶ **TIP** All prenatal multivitamin tablets contain around 1000 micrograms (1 mg) of folic acid, so you are well covered if you take one a day.

② Stop Drinking Alcohol

Fetal Alcohol Spectrum Disorder (FASD) is the leading cause of *preventable* brain damage in infants and children. The great beauty of planning your pregnancy is that you can take steps to avoid exposures to alcohol in plenty of time to ensure that your baby is safeguarded against its harmful effects.

Unfortunately, not all women (and their babies) are so lucky. Nearly 50% of all pregnancies are unplanned. What's more, nearly 50% of women of childbearing age consume alcohol in varying amounts. This means that nearly 25% of all babies will be exposed to some level of alcohol before they are born. What that means to their growth and development will depend in large part on the amount of the prenatal exposure.

If a lot of alcohol will produce the worst harm, and less alcohol will produce different effects, what (you may ask) is a safe amount to drink during pregnancy? The answer is, we just don't know. That's why the most prudent choice when planning your pregnancy is to avoid alcohol entirely.

▶ **TIP** If avoiding alcohol is a challenge for you, try to get help. The Motherisk Alcohol Helpline at (877) 327-4636 can answer questions and refer you to programs and services.

③ Stop Cigarette Smoking

Before pregnancy you should stop smoking. Smoking in pregnancy may decrease the baby's birth weight and increase the risk of stillbirth (fetal death after 20 weeks of gestation) and prematurity (baby born before 37 weeks of pregnancy). It also increases your risk for miscarriage. Last, but not least, smoking in pregnancy is associated with Sudden Infant Death Syndrome (SIDS) or 'crib death', where infants die during their sleep.

▶ **TIP** If you're having trouble kicking the smoking habit, you may want to think about getting help. Talk to your doctor. Nicotine replacement therapy (nicotine patch, gum, or spray) or Zyban (bupropion) tablets may be right for you. Both methods have been shown in controlled randomized trials to be effective in smoking cessation.

④ Immunize Against Dangerous Infectious Diseases

When you plan pregnancy, you should ensure that you are immunized against several viruses that are dangerous for the unborn baby. The most important one is rubella (German measles). If you have not had rubella before, or if you were not immunized, your unborn baby will not be protected. If the virus of rubella attacks the fetus, the result may be Congenital Rubella Syndrome, which is characterized by deafness, mental retardation, and other effects, such as heart anomalies in the child. Vaccination against rubella is crucial because your other young children may contract the illness in daycare or school, or you may contract it from other young children (neighbors, friends, family). If you work with children (as a teacher or care-taker), it is even more important to be vaccinated.

The other virus that can adversely affect the fetus and for which there is a vaccine is chickenpox (varicella). When con-tracted by pregnant women who did not have chickenpox before, a small percent of unborn babies (1% to 2%) may con-tract fetal varicella syndrome, which affects the brain, eyes, and limb formation. Here, too, you can get the vaccine from your doctor after a blood test that shows you are not immune.

▶ **TIP** For more information on vaccinations for chicken pox, influenza, and other infectious diseases, see Chapter 11, "Medical Conditions and Infections."

⑤ Seek Preconception Genetic Counseling

If there is a history in your family of children born with con-genital malformations or developmental delays, either your own children or those of your siblings, or the siblings of the father of your unborn baby, this is the time for genetic coun-seling. Your doctor can refer you for counseling. Genetic counseling usually involves a detailed assessment of your medical, obstetric, and family history, as well as various labo-ratory tests.

▶ **TIP** Some important genetic tests are described in Chapter 4, "Assessing Risk."

⑥ Treat Drug or Chemical Dependencies

If you are chemically dependent on or addicted to a recreational drug, such as cocaine or marijuana, it is advisable to seek addiction counseling and treatment before pregnancy. Drugs of abuse may affect your baby directly by entering the baby's body, or indirectly by affecting your health and/or your ability to care for your baby when born. Remember too that drug dependence is not limited to the use of 'street drugs' but may also involve common medications such as pain relievers.

▶ **TIP** Some of the consequences of drug abuse during pregnancy are described in Chapter 9, "Alcohol, Smoking, and Drug Abuse." The Motherisk Alcohol and Substance Use Helpline may be able to help with information and referrals to counseling at (877) 327-4636.

⑦ Avoid Workplace Exposures to Dangerous Chemicals

If you are employed in a workplace where you may be exposed to chemicals, it is important to seek counseling about what is safe and what is not. Exposure to chemical solvents and heavy metals can pose a risk to your baby. The ones you have probably heard the most about are carbon monoxide, formaldehyde, lead, mercury, and organic solvents. There are others.

▶ **TIP** For more information on ways of protecting yourself from exposure to dangerous chemicals, see Chapter 10, "Chemical and Radiation Exposures."

⑧ Seek Proper Treatment of Maternal Medical Conditions

If you suffer from a medical condition, this is the time to ensure that you are treated well with medications that are safe for the fetus. While this book contains a lot of details on medications and medical conditions, it cannot — and indeed does not intend to — replace the advice of your health-care provider. You should discuss whether pregnancy will affect your medical condition and vice versa (whether your medical condition will affect the pregnancy).

▶ **TIP** Chapter 11, "Medical Conditions and Infections," covers some of the more common chronic maternal medical conditions and how to reduce risk.

CHAPTER ONE

Introduction

Last December, I sought your help regarding a couple of tranquilizers I had taken within the first few weeks of my pregnancy.... As a result of your advice, my husband and I are the ecstatic parents of a beautiful, healthy baby girl. I cannot thank you enough.

— Motherisk Caller

When it comes to pregnancy, it seems everybody's an expert. Family, friends, neighbors — even total strangers — all have advice for the pregnant woman. And though all of it may be entirely well meaning, very little of it is likely to be clinically sound — especially when it comes to the use of medications and the exposure to potentially toxic substances during pregnancy. That's why when there's a question about the risk or safety of medications, chemicals, alcohol, infectious disease, or other exposures during pregnancy, the only good advice is to consult your physician and a teratogen information center.

Pregnancy Paranoia

Teratogens are substances or environmental factors that can cause birth defects. In order for a drug, chemical, or infection to be considered a teratogen, there must be substantive evidence that being exposed to it causes birth defects.

In a recent article in *The New York Times*, several concerned pregnant women listed among suspected teratogens underwire bras, thongs, hair dryers, acrylic nails, cellphones, chocolate mousse, bikini waxes, farmed salmon, blue cheese, hair dye, Botox, deli meats, champagne, tanning beds, hot dogs, albacore tuna … and more. Some of their fears were well founded in evidence-based medical research; others were old wives' tales and urban legends.

Part of the purpose of this book is to sort out the facts from the myths. A related purpose is to counsel women who are considering conceiving or who are now pregnant. Not all exposures to teratogens pose the same risk — in fact, there are many that are unlikely to cause harm. What's more, a woman who has relied on medications to control medical conditions, such as hypertension and depression, may do more harm than good by suddenly going off her medication once she learns that she is pregnant.

The key to a safe pregnancy, then, is sound counseling based on up-to-date, evidence-based research.

FACT ✓ **Thalidomide Tragedy**

Perhaps the most well-known and feared teratogen is thalidomide. The use of thalidomide for the treatment of morning sickness caused major malformations among nearly 10,000 exposed children born in the 1950s and early 1960s. The thalidomide tragedy (as many came to call it) was so frightening that it was not long before *every* medication, environmental exposure, and virus in pregnancy was viewed with alarm.

The Motherisk Program

Since 1985 Motherisk, a program of The Hospital for Sick Children in Toronto, has offered sound counseling based on up-to-date, evidence-based research. The only teratogen information program in Canada, Motherisk is also one of the largest programs of its kind in the world. To date, the program has counseled more than 400,000 women.

Synonymous with 'motherhood', Motherisk is an invaluable international resource and service. Every day, Motherisk counselors answer calls from hundreds of women and their doctors, seeking important information about the safety or risk of common medications, drugs, medicinal plants, chemicals, infections, and other agents that might affect their unborn children. Some of the questions are easy — our information reassuring. Others are a lot harder.

As you might guess, not every question has a ready answer. Each day, women and their doctors are faced with new drugs and exposures that simply have not been studied for their potential risk to the unborn. If they are to make informed choices that will affect them and their children for life, mothers-to-be need to know.

That's why at Motherisk, laboratory and population research is a vital part of what we do. Right now, pioneering research is underway to establish the risks of diseases and their treatment during pregnancy, to determine the safety of herbal products, and to establish once and for all the devastating effects of acute morning sickness in pregnancy — just to name a few.

MOTHERISK MANDATE

1. To provide authoritative information and guidance to pregnant and breastfeeding women and their health-care providers regarding the fetal risks associated with drug, chemical, infection, disease, and/or radiation exposure during pregnancy and lactation.

2. To research unanswered questions on the safety of drugs, chemicals, infection, disease, and radiation during pregnancy and lactation.

3. To maintain a vital training and educational program in the areas of reproductive and developmental toxicology at the undergraduate, graduate, and postgraduate levels.

MOTHERISK HELPLINES, WEBSITE, & ON-LINE FORUMS

Motherisk counselors are available weekdays from 9:00 a.m. to 5:00 p.m. (EST) and operate the following helplines.

Motherisk Main Line
(416) 813-6780
For information about the risk or safety of prescription and over-the-counter drugs, herbal products, chemicals, x-rays, chronic disease, and infections during pregnancy. This is a toll call to our Toronto call center. Callers may have to wait up to 10 minutes to speak to a counselor.

In the evening and on the weekends when Motherisk counselors are not on duty, a series of recorded messages provide basic information on some of the most frequently asked questions about exposures during pregnancy and while breastfeeding. Callers can hear those messages by dialing (416) 813-6780.

Alcohol and Substance Use Helpline
(877) 327-4636
For information about the fetal effects of alcohol, nicotine, and drugs like marijuana, cocaine, and ecstasy.

Nausea and Vomiting of Pregnancy Helpline
(800) 436-8477
For information on morning sickness and how to treat it.

HIV and HIV Treatment in Pregnancy
(888) 246-5840
For information about the possible effects of HIV and HIV treatment during pregnancy.

Motherisk Website
www.motherisk.org
The Motherisk website is another very good resource. Each month more than 25,000 website visitors search the site for published research on a broad range of medications and other exposures. The Motherisk website also features two on-line forums that answer visitors' specific questions. The Nausea and Vomiting of Pregnancy Forum fields patients' questions about morning sickness and how to cope, and the Cancer in Pregnancy Forum considers questions submitted by physicians on the treatment of pregnant women with cancer.

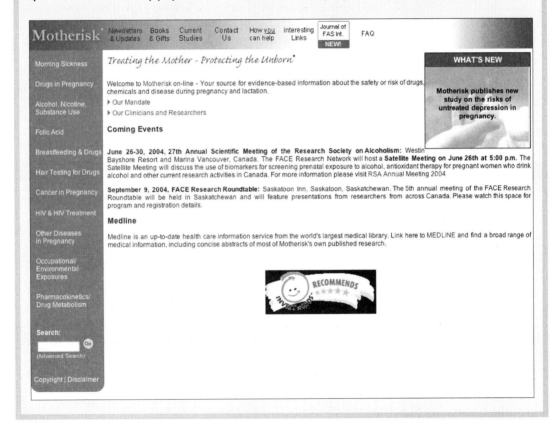

Results
The research, education, and counseling that we're doing are paying off. Since 1985, Motherisk's multidisciplinary team of physicians, pharmacologists, toxicologists, geneticists, pharmacists, epidemiologists, and psychiatrists has achieved the following:

• Delivered authoritative and often reassuring information about the safety of important drugs for women with chronic conditions, such as epilepsy, arthritis, and depression.

- Disproved traditional 'wisdom' that debilitating morning sickness is "all in a woman's head" and advocated safe and effective treatment.
- Established the Province of Ontario's first diagnostic program for Fetal Alcohol Spectrum Disorder.
- Created Canada's first pilot program to diagnose and treat chicken pox in pregnancy.
- Helped hundreds of women avoid termination of wanted pregnancies.

This book contains much of the information that Motherisk counselors share with nearly 200 callers each day. In so doing, we hope to help ensure rational treatment for women during pregnancy and while breastfeeding — and a healthy start for newborn children.

We invite you to consult this book as a reference throughout your pregnancy and once your baby is born and nursing.

Calling a Teratogen Service Helpline

Motherisk receives approximately 3,000 telephone calls each month from Canadians and Americans. Combined with e-mails and visits to the Motherisk website, these calls to Motherisk helplines demonstrate the growing sensitivity among not only pregnant and breastfeeding women but also their physicians regarding the safety/risk of drugs, chemicals, radiation, and infections.

Motherisk Helpline counselors answer these calls and e-mail inquiries. Motherisk hears from women planning their pregnancy, pregnant women, and breastfeeding women, as well as their partners, physicians, pharmacists, and other health professionals. Calls are also received from the general public and from the healthcare media – newspapers, magazines, radio, television — seeking authoritative information on the safety of new drugs and therapies during pregnancy and breastfeeding.

Counselor's Role and Referrals

Each call is handled by a Motherisk counselor — a trained, information specialist with a background in clinical pharmacology. With each question, Motherisk counselors decide whether the caller should be referred for a clinic appointment or to the physician on call, or whether there is appropriate information that can be shared with the caller at the time of the call. The counselor conducts a careful interview to determine all potential risk factors before providing the latest, evidence-based information available. The counselor also completes a detailed Telephone Call Report Form. Daily summary sheets are retained for reference and follow-up.

Each week pregnant women are scheduled for the Motherisk clinic following exposure to known or suspected teratogens, new drugs about which little is known, chronic drug therapy, or drugs of abuse. Still others are referred to the Motherisk clinic to address their extreme anxiety.

BE PREPARED

To make the most of your call to Motherisk or other teratogen center, make sure that you have some basic information handy before you dial. If you are calling about the use of a medication during pregnancy, know the exact name of the drug and why you are taking it. For example, if you are taking Tylenol for a cough or cold, be prepared to tell the counselor which one you are taking (there are about 10 different Tylenol brands of cough and cold medication on the market). The best thing is to have the medicine bottle or prescription in your hand when you call. That way, you will be able to provide important information about what the drug contains and how much you are taking. If you are calling about a workplace exposure, it is not enough to tell the Motherisk counselor where you work or what kind of work you do. Know the name of the chemical or other agent that you are concerned about.

Risk Assessment and Management

How do we judge the safety or risk of exposure to drugs, chemicals, and infections during pregnancy and breastfeeding? This is a question of 'risk assessment and management'. In fact, it's something we all do every day. For example, when driving a car along a residential street, we face the risk that a child or the neighbor's cat may suddenly dart across the street. We manage that risk by driving more slowly. But we don't quit driving down all residential streets simply because that risk exists.

The same can be said about medications, chemicals, and infections during pregnancy and breastfeeding. Some substances pose a greater risk than others, but that doesn't mean you must avoid all important medication, quit your job, or stop treatment of a disease condition for the full 9 months of your pregnancy.

We live in an imperfect world. There are no guarantees in life — or pregnancy. That said, there is plenty of available, evidence-based information that can help us make sound choices.

So when it comes to determining whether or not to take a particular medication during pregnancy, for example, the best you and your doctor can (and must) do is balance the therapeutic benefit to you against what is known about the potential effect on the fetus. What's more, you must be sure that this balancing act is not tipped by misinformation, undue fear of unproven risks, or pressure from uninformed sources.

SAFETY/RISK ❖ Consult with Your Doctor

Before making any decision based on the information you find in this book, be sure to consult with your doctor. The information contained here is not meant to replace the advice your physician or other health-care providers. Always be sure to consult your physician before taking medications or changing any current treatment.

Using this Book

This book begins by raising and answering a series of frequently asked questions about safety/risk in pregnancy and breastfeeding, then expands on each answer in successive chapters. Within chapters, you will find quick reference charts and lists of medications, chemicals, and infections 'graded' according to their safety/risk. We also provide a comprehensive Index identifying all medications, chemicals, and infections mentioned in the book for quick reference. If you are especially worried about any one medication, chemical, or infection, you might start with the Index.

RISK GRADES

Several health regulatory agencies have developed different ways to express 'safety' and 'risk' when evaluating drugs taken during pregnancy and breastfeeding. The most widely used categories have been developed by the United States Federal Drug Administration (FDA), with 'A' assigned to the safest drugs and 'X' assigned to drugs contraindicated in pregnancy. However, this system has been criticized because it is confusing and often inaccurate. The FDA is currently in the process of changing this system entirely.

At Motherisk, we have established a system for grading the risk of prescription and over-the-counter drugs in pregnancy, ranging from 'Safe' to 'Unsafe'. This does not mean that everything that is not deemed 'Safe' is 'Unsafe' and must be avoided during pregnancy. There are *degrees of safety* that should be considered, especially if the medication is important for the health and well-being of the mother. These degrees of safety are vital to balancing the benefit and the risk of various medications.

Safe

Safe means that a convincing and authoritative body of scientific evidence, accumulated over time, through sound scientific research, shows no adverse effects on the fetus.

Probably Safe

Probably Safe means that there is no evidence the drug is dangerous to the fetus and that the information showing it to be safe is rather large. Here, the benefit/risk assessment will be weighted, in most cases, in favor of using the medication.

Possibly Safe

Possibly Safe means that there is no evidence that the drug is dangerous for the fetus, but the information showing it to be safe is limited. By 'limited' we mean that only a few studies have been published in the medical literature, or the studies that are available do not meet all of the rigorous standards of critical scientific appraisal.

Unsafe

Unsafe means that there is evidence to show that the medication may cause harmful effects during pregnancy or during a particular trimester of pregnancy. This does not mean that the harm is certain to happen in each and every case of exposure, but there is enough risk of harm to justify careful use or avoidance in pregnancy.

Unknown or Unclear

Unknown or *Unclear* means that there is simply not enough reliable information for us to be able to determine safety or risk in pregnancy. This may change over time as evidence-based research uncovers more information about the effects of these drugs.

CHAPTER TWO

Frequently Asked Questions

I desperately needed help when I found out I was pregnant. First, because of the "surprise" and second because I was undergoing treatment for Rosacea and was taking antibiotics.... Then I called Motherisk. The calm person who answered my call that day asked me a few questions and was able to confirm that all would be well with the fetus due to the stage I was at and the amount of drugs I had taken. I went on to give birth to a beautiful, healthy baby boy just before Christmas — we called him Deaven (from heaven!) and he's been a constant joy to all our lives. Thank you, thank you, thank you.

— ***Motherisk Caller***

The following *broad* questions and *brief* answers describe the kind of information that Motherisk teratogen counselors are regularly called upon to provide. They also define the organizing principle for this book, in that each question corresponds to a chapter in the book. As you read on, you will learn much more about each topic and the many factors and considerations that go into providing the right answers.

Assessing Risk

Q How can I ensure that my pregnancy is 100% risk free?

A The short answer is, you can't. But that's still no reason to be alarmed. The vast majority of children born are normal and healthy. However, in the general population, between one and five out of every 100 children born will have major malformations. This 'baseline risk' is a fact of life, even for the woman who manages to avoid medications, chemicals, infections, and other exposures during pregnancy. Fortunately, many of these malformations can be corrected through surgery. For example, many malformations of the heart can be corrected by surgery. However, the one area where we still do not have good medical solutions to congenital malformation is brain development.

▶ **LOOK AHEAD** Tests for determining risk are described in Chapter 4, "Assessing Risk."

Morning Sickness

Q Does everyone get morning sickness and how long does it usually last?

A Morning sickness, also known as nausea and vomiting of pregnancy (NVP), affects up to 80% of pregnant women. If you are pregnant and suffering with morning sickness, you are definitely not alone. Though usually limited to the first 7 to 12 weeks of pregnancy, approximately 20% of pregnant women experience morning sickness for a longer period of time. Some women may suffer until the end of the pregnancy.

▶ **LOOK AHEAD** You can read more about morning sickness, its treatment, and how to cope in Chapter 5, "Morning Sickness." Another great resource is the on-line Motherisk NVP Forum. Go to www.motherisk.org/forum and post a question for the Motherisk NVP counselor — or read what others have asked.

Prescription Drugs

Q *Should a woman avoid all medications while she is pregnant?*

A Although there is good reason for therapeutic caution during pregnancy, there are instances where the benefits of continuing drug therapy outweigh the risks. Careful 'risk/benefit analysis' may determine that a woman taking medication under a doctor's supervision should continue to do so. Some of the best examples are the proper use of medication to treat seizure disorders and the use of antidepressants to control mood disorders common in pregnancy.

▶ **LOOK AHEAD** A comprehensive list of medications, evaluated for their degree of risk, is provided in Chapter 6, "Prescription Drugs."

Over-the-Counter Medications

Q *Can I take over-the-counter drugs while I'm pregnant?*

A We'll have much more to say on this topic later, but for now suffice it to say that some over-the-counter drugs (OTCs) can be used safely, while others cannot. The most important thing to remember is "Don't Self-Prescribe." Talk to you doctor before you take anything during your 9 months (or more) of pregnancy.

▶ **LOOK AHEAD** For an evaluation of over-the-counter medications for such common illnesses and conditions as colds, allergies, and skin irritations, see Chapter 7, "Over-the-Counter Medications."

Herbal Products and Natural Medicines

Q *Are herbal medicines such as echinacea, St. John's wort, and others safe to use during pregnancy?*

A A study conducted in 1996 showed that nearly 60% of women surveyed believed that herbal remedies were helpful in preventing and treating illness. Thousands of so-called natural medicines are consumed by women of reproductive age, many of whom may wrongly assume that 'natural' automatically means 'safe.' The truth is that little is known about the risk or safety of herbal medicines, since manufacturers of herbal medicines, unlike the makers of pharmaceutical drugs, are not bound by legislation to test their safety in all jurisdictions. What's more, most medicinal plants contain scores of active ingredients in concentrations that may differ from crop to crop and even within a single plant.

This problem of quality and purity is being addressed by the Natural Health Products Directorate (NHPD) division of Health Canada, the Food and Drug Administration (FDA) agency in the United States, and similar regulatory bodies in Europe. At Motherisk, we are also examining herbal medicines one by one and have made important findings on a limited number of them. There is still much more research to be done in this particular area of teratology.

▶ **LOOK AHEAD** Chapter 8 includes a guide to common herbal products and what researchers have determined regarding their safety.

Alcohol, Cigarette Smoking, and Drug Abuse

Q *Is it true that a single drink during pregnancy can harm the baby?*

A Researchers still have not established how much alcohol can be consumed safely during pregnancy. As a result, a safe amount of alcohol in pregnancy is not known. It is very unlikely, though, that a single drink before you knew you were pregnant could damage your unborn baby. You should avoid drinking when you know that you are pregnant. If you are planning a pregnancy, plan to quit before you get pregnant.

Q I'm planning a pregnancy. How important is it that I quit smoking?

A It is very important. When compared to babies of non-smokers, those whose mothers smoke tend to be smaller and more often premature. They have a two to three times higher risk of stillbirth (death in the womb) and of crib death (Sudden Infant Death Syndrome or SIDS) after birth. Children who grow up with smoking parents have a much higher risk of developing asthma, bronchitis, and ear infections, most probably due to the irritating effects of some of the chemicals emitted in cigarette smoke.

Q What are the effects of cocaine use in pregnancy?

A Studies have shown that cocaine exposure during pregnancy is associated with serious health hazards, such as intrauterine growth restriction, prematurity, stillbirth, perinatal complications, and abruption of the placenta, probably due to increased blood pressure caused by cocaine. The bleeding that occurs in an abruption can cause acute decrease in blood supply to the fetus, and this in turn can cause serious fetal damage or even death.

▶ **LOOK AHEAD** Chapter 9 has much more information about alcohol, cigarette smoke, and recreational drugs. Also see Chapter 14, "Breastfeeding and Drugs," for the effects of alcohol on breastfeeding children.

Chemical and Radiation Exposures

Q Is it safe to continue to work throughout my pregnancy if there are chemicals in my workplace?

A This is a difficult question. Generally, if you are working with or around chemicals, you need to know the facts about that workplace exposure. It is likely that your employer keeps data safety sheets describing the limit of safe exposure for an adult. The employer may also measure and record the amount of the chemicals that are in the air where you work. You should be able to discuss this data with your company's occupational health nurse or other corporate representative. Remember, though, that available safety data is usually limited to the effect of the chemical on an adult — not an unborn baby. Still, before you decide to start a new job or quit your old one, consult a teratogen counselor for the latest information on workplace and environmental exposures.

▶ **LOOK AHEAD** Consult Chapter 10, "Chemical and Radiation Exposures," for information on specific exposures.

Medical Conditions and Infections

Q *If I get sick during pregnancy, how will this affect my baby?*

A Exposure to certain infectious diseases, such as varicella (chicken pox) and rubella (German measles), pose a risk to your unborn baby. Certain chronic conditions and their treatment may also increase reproductive risks. What's more, certain chronic conditions, such as depression, can harm your newborn baby by impairing your ability to care for your newborn. That's why it's important to look after yourself before and after pregnancy, and seek the treatment you need.

Q *I'm a schoolteacher and 3 months pregnant. The children in my school are coming down with chicken pox. My mother does not remember whether I had chicken pox as a child, and I am worried because I heard the infection could affect my baby. Is this true?*

A About 70% of all women who do not recall having had chicken pox (varicella) when they were young did in fact have it. You can confirm this by measuring antibodies in your blood. However, once you are pregnant and have been in contact with children with chicken pox, measuring antibodies in your blood may take too long. Your doctor should therefore give you antibodies called VZIG (varicella zoster immune globulins) to decrease the risk of fetal infection.

▶ **LOOK AHEAD** A comprehensive guide to the risks associated with such medical conditions and infections as diabetes, cancer, and heart disease is presented in Chapter 11, "Medical Conditions and Infections."

Food, Nutritional Supplements, and Dieting

Q Should I be supplementing my diet in any way?

A Some of the most exciting news in medical science these days is what we have learned about the prevention of neural tube defects, such as spina bifida and anencephaly. We now have concrete evidence that these conditions can be prevented if women take enough folic acid before and while they are pregnant. Folic acid is a vitamin found in foods like dark green vegetables, liver, and lentils. It is also contained in prenatal vitamin supplements.

Q Are there foods I should avoid during pregnancy?

A Though pregnancy is a special time for most women, there is no reason why ordinary, everyday common sense won't apply to most choices about diet and food. Prepare and cook your food well (to avoid toxoplasmosis), follow a balanced diet plan such as the USDA Food Guide Pyramid or Canada's Food Guide to Healthy Eating, and you should be fine. Fish should be eaten in moderation to control the risk of exposure to mercury, but it doesn't have to be eliminated from your diet. After all, seafood is an important source of essential nutrients and fatty acids.

▶ **LOOK AHEAD** Chapter 12 has more advice about foods, diets, and supplements.

Work, Exercise, and Sex

Q *I work full time in a factory where I spend a lot of time on my feet. Can I continue to work while I'm pregnant?*

A In most cases, women can continue working safely throughout their pregnancy. There are, however, certain risks that you should be aware of and avoid. If there is a risk of chemical or radiation exposure, you'll want to learn as much as you can about what that might be. You will also want to avoid heavy lifting, standing for long periods of time, and working more than 40 hours per week. Let your employer know that you are pregnant, in case you need to make small changes to improve the safety of your workplace for the next 9 months. Most employers will respond positively — after all, a healthy workplace is good for business too.

▶ **LOOK AHEAD** For more information about work, exercise, sex, and related lifestyle risks, see Chapter 13.

Breastfeeding and Drugs

Q *Once my baby is born and I'm breastfeeding, do I still have to be cautious about the use of medications?*

A Though many drugs are quite safe for a mother to take while nursing her child, there are several for which safety during breastfeeding is not well defined and may pose a risk to the infant.

▶ **LOOK AHEAD** Drugs that are contraindicated or should be used with caution by lactating women are described in Chapter 14, "Breastfeeding and Drugs."

CHAPTER THREE

Research Questions and (Some) Answers

I would like to thank you all for the support and peace of mind you gave me during my first pregnancy. I called regarding antibiotics that I took ... before discovering my pregnancy. Your knowledge and compassion restored my sanity. I hope to never require your services again, but I am thankful that your organization exists for other mothers.

— *Motherisk Caller*

Pregnant women are not the only people at Motherisk who ask difficult questions. So does our team of medical researchers. Preliminary answers to some of these questions give us a better understanding of the kind of risks involved in pregnancy.

While we can provide brief answers to these questions here, you may want to consult the Motherisk website at www.motherisk.org for an extensive record of research reports written on these subjects.

Congenital Malformations

Q *When do medications, chemicals, and infections cause malformations?*

A Primarily during the first trimester (12-14 weeks) of pregnancy when all of the baby's organs are forming. After the first trimester of pregnancy, the tiny organs and limbs continue to develop and grow. The small fingers become bigger, but no new fingers are formed. The only organ that continues to develop throughout (and even after) pregnancy is the brain.

Some teratogens interfere with the normal process of development, causing organs to develop incompletely, or in a wrong way. For example, several antiepileptic drugs can cause neural tube defects.

FACT ✔ First Trimester Dangers

Most drugs, chemicals, and infections that cause congenital malformations will do so during the first trimester of pregnancy, when they can interfere with the normal development of organs.

Q What is a neural tube defect?

A Neural tube defects are caused by the incomplete closure of the neural crest (the original nervous system). A child with a neural tube defect (NTD) can be born with an incomplete spinal cord or brain. For example, the drug Depakene (valproic acid) causes this malformation in about 2% of exposed pregnancies, while the drug Tegretol (carbamazepine) causes it in 1% of exposed pregnancies. However, the time at which the exposure occurred is very important. Because the neural tube is normally closed at 4 weeks of pregnancy, Depakene and Tegretol can interfere with that process only very early in pregnancy. That means that if a pregnant woman starts taking Tegretol at 12 weeks of pregnancy, the medication will not interfere with neural tube closure.

Q What risks may follow in the second and third trimester?

A Since the brain continues to develop throughout pregnancy, medication and chemicals that adversely affect brain development may cause harm even in late pregnancy. For example, alcohol may cause fetal damage at any point in pregnancy, including late pregnancy. The virus that causes Fifth Disease may cause the breakdown of fetal blood (hemolysis) and thus may endanger the life of the fetus, even though it does not cause any malformation.

ACE inhibitors, such as enalapril, provide another example. These drugs are widely used for hypertension (high blood pressure). When taken during pregnancy, ACE inhibitors can cause the fetal kidneys to shut down, so that the baby is born with non-functioning kidneys. This effect occurs in late pregnancy. That is why drugs such as enalapril, lisinopril, and others like them should not be used in late pregnancy. Other drugs that are 'contraindicated' (not to be used) in pregnancy will be discussed throughout this book.

FACT ✔ Fetal Organs and Tissues

A medication, chemical, or infection may also damage the unborn without interfering with organogenesis (cellular formation). Such teratogens affect fetal organs or tissues that are already formed.

Q What risks may follow after birth?

A Sudden Infant Death Syndrome (SIDS) or crib death happens when an apparently healthy baby, typically in the first months of life, goes to sleep at night and dies during sleep. In order to be diagnosed as SIDS, no other condition can be found, such as heart malformation, lung infection, or brain anomalies. SIDS happens more often among boys than girls, and more often among twins and other multiple pregnancies than single births. The peak of the condition is at around 4 to 6 months of life.

Extensive research has not yet identified exactly why SIDS happens, but studies of 'near SIDS' children and repeated events of near SIDS in the same babies have shown that these children have prolonged apnea (lack of breathing).

Cigarette smoking during pregnancy and smoking after pregnancy are strongly associated with SIDS. Babies of smokers have three to four times more risk of SIDS. The other strong causative factor for SIDS is the method of sleeping. Sleeping prone (on the belly) bears the highest risk for SIDS. Sleeping supine (on the back) has the lowest risk. Sleeping on the side has an intermediate risk.

Teratogen Transfer

Q How are teratogens transmitted from mother to fetus?

A Although it was once thought that the placenta (the organ that develops in the uterus during pregnancy and serves to nourish the fetus) formed a protective barrier against all harmful agents, we now know better. At Motherisk, we conduct 'placental perfusion' studies to identify those substances and compounds that can cross the placenta and in what amount. What we are learning is opening up new therapeutic approaches to delivering important medications to the fetus through the pregnant woman. In years to come, we will see an increase in the number of therapies available to the caregiver or clinician aimed at assisting the unborn child.

FACT ✔ Dose and Timing

Many agents in the pregnant woman's circulatory system cross the placenta to reach the fetus. The important questions are how much may have reached the fetus (dose), and at what point in the fetus's development (timing).

Unknown Mechanisms

Q How do teratogens affect the fetus?

A Medications, chemicals, infections, and other maternal exposures during pregnancy can affect the fetus in a variety of ways. We have already described the way some drugs can interfere with organ development (organogenesis), while others can affect the fetus *after* organ development but *before* birth. What's more, damaging effects may vary from fetus to fetus.

Understanding precisely how teratogens operate to produce these effects is a difficult and important science that seeks to answer many intriguing questions. For example, one of the great mysteries of Fetal Alcohol Spectrum Syndrome is that out of 100 fetuses exposed to heavy drinking, only two to five will sustain the full-blown syndrome, 10% to 30% will exhibit a partial syndrome, and the rest will escape the major signs of brain toxicity. What saves this group of babies? Is it that different placentae handle alcohol differently? Or are different fetuses able to cope in various ways with this toxin?

Similarly, why is it that more than two-thirds of infants of HIV-infected mothers never show signs of infection? What protects them? Is it the amount of infection existing in the mother's body or the amount of antibodies produced by the mother? When does the virus cross the human placenta? If evidence shows that cesarean section in HIV-positive women decreases the positivity of infants, can we say with scientific certainty that most babies are infected during their passage through the birth canal?

FETAL ORGAN DEVELOPMENT (WEEKLY)

WEEK 1	WEEK 2	WEEK 3	WEEK 4	WEEK 5	WEEK 6
	Common Site of Teratogen Action				
Not Susceptible to Teratogenesis (Week 1–2) ⟶		Major Congenital Anomalies (Week 3–8) ————————————————			
		Neural Tube Defects ————————————————⟶			
		Truncus Ateriosus/Atrial Septal Defect/Ventricular Septal Defect			
			Amelia/Miromelia ———⟶	Upper Limb	
			Amelia/Miromelia ———⟶	Lower Limb	
				Cleft Lip ——————⟶	
			Low-set Malformed Ears and Deafness ———		
			Microphthalmia, Cataracts, Glaucoma ———		
				⟵	
					Cleft Palate

The answers to these and other 'variability in response' questions are still unknown. Yet finding the answers could help save lives and treat those who do not escape harm. Motherisk is committed to finding these answers.

RESOURCES

For current research into these and other questions, be sure to consult the Motherisk website at www.motherisk.org and the Organization of Teratology Information Services (OTIS) at www.otispregnancy.org.

This fetal development chart illustrates how the organs develop from Week 1 to Week 38 of pregnancy. The effects of chemicals and other exposures during pregnancy will depend in large part on which organs are developing at the time of exposure.

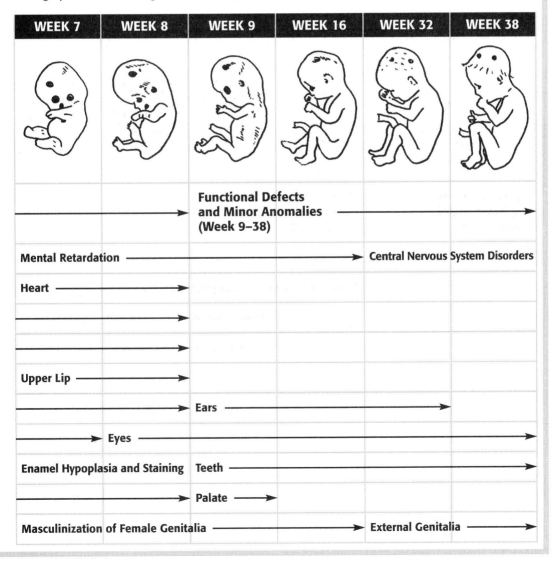

CHAPTER FOUR

Assessing Risk

What a privilege it is to have access to such a wealth of information! Congratulations to the Motherisk program for your web site. I am now in my 16th week of my pregnancy and I found the information on your site to be very useful for both myself and my husband.

— **Motherisk Website Visitor**

Prenatal Screening and Diagnostic Tests

Genes are the pieces of DNA that define each person's physical, mental, and psychological makeup. They are packaged in 46 chromosomes that reside in each cell of our body. Half of our genes come from our mother and half from our father. When something wrong happens in our genes, the result may be a congenital malformation.

The science of prenatal testing is developing rapidly. *Screening* tests during early pregnancy can alert a woman to a potential defect in congenital genetic conditions. In most developed and developing countries, pregnant women are offered, as part of regular follow-up, blood tests and ultrasound to predict the likelihood that the unborn child has a congenital condition, such as Down Syndrome and neural tube defects.

FACT ✔ **Detecting Malformations**

Out of 100 babies born, between one and five will have a major congenital malformation that can often be recognized through prenatal tests.

Depending on the results of the *screening* tests, the woman and her caregiver may decide to proceed with further *diagnostic* tests (such as amniocentesis and cordocentesis) to confirm whether her unborn child is affected.

These prenatal tests can be a source of important information. For example, if you have already had a child with a genetic condition (such as cystic fibrosis or hemophilia), tests of cells of the fetus obtained during amniocentesis will detect whether your unborn baby is also affected.

SAFETY/RISK ❖ Important Decision

Whether or not to proceed with prenatal genetic testing is an important decision that should be made with all the facts before you. The following pages describe some of the more widely used procedures, how they work, what they can detect, their possible risks to the fetus, and who might be a good candidate for such testing. However, if you have had a child with a genetic disorder, or if there are individuals in your family with congenital problems (e.g., hearing loss, mental retardation), you should ask to be referred to a genetic service in your area. Genetic and maternal-fetal specialists are the professionals best qualified to conduct all the required tests and, hopefully, help prevent your unborn baby from having the same congenital problem.

Maternal Tests

The prenatal tests described here and a detailed ultrasound at 16 to 18 weeks of pregnancy can detect many, though not all, congenital malformations in the fetus.

Blood Tests

Maternal blood tests during pregnancy predict certain congenital malformations and conditions, such as neural tube defects and Down Syndrome. These tests, alone or in combination, predict these malformations during pregnancy.

Blood tests also predict congenital conditions that may have been caused by the use of certain drugs during pregnancy. For example, a pregnant woman who is treated with Tegretol (carbamazepine) or Depakene (valproic acid) may run the risk of having a child with a neural tube defect, such as spina bifida. Blood tests can help rule out this risk. The numerical values of these tests change from one place to the other. This means that normal ranges may be expressed in different ways. Your caregiver will discuss the ranges with you and where you are within that range.

Blood tests also measure the levels of different medications in a woman's system. This is important in those cases where it is necessary to continue a medication even during pregnancy in order to treat properly certain serious medical conditions. The course of treatment should be monitored because the ability of the body in a pregnant woman to eliminate medications may increase as the pregnancy progresses. As a result, a daily dose that was adequate before pregnancy may not be sufficient in late pregnancy. For medications where routine blood levels are conducted, it is important to monitor levels in late pregnancy.

Properly conducted, a maternal blood test should pose no risk to the unborn child.

RISK OF DOWN SYNDROME
and All Chromosome Abnormalities at Different Maternal Ages

It is well established that as a woman gets older, her risk of having a child with certain chromosome abnormalities, including Down Syndrome, increases. Prenatal diagnosis for this syndrome is usually offered to women who are over 35 at the expected date of delivery and to women in risk as indicated by other screening tests. Prenatal diagnosis is also offered to mothers who have had a previous child with a chromosomal abnormality.

Maternal Age at Delivery (years)	Risk of Down Syndrome	Risk of All Chromosome Abnormalities
25	1/1270	1/480
30	1/970	1/390
35	1/330	1/180
36	1/255	1/150
37	1/205	1/125
38	1/155	1/100
39	1/125	1/80
40	1/95	1/65
41	1/73	1/50
42	1/55	1/40
43	1/45	1/30
44	1/35	1/24
45	1/28	1/19

MEDICATION LEVELS (CONCENTRATIONS) IN THE BLOOD

This table lists medications for which levels are routinely tested in the blood. Appropriate levels are critical in women who have undergone organ transplant and have been treated with cyclosporine or tacrolimus. They are also important for women who are treated with lithium for bipolar mood disorder; women treated with digoxin, quinidine, amiodarone, and other drugs for cardiac conditions; and women treated with carbamazepine or phenytoin for epilepsy — to name just a few.

Heart Drugs	Digoxin, Disopyramide, Lidocaine, Procainamide, Quinidine
Antibiotics	Gentamicin, Tobramycin, Amikacin
Antiepileptics	Carbamazepine, Phenytoin, Phenobarbital, Valproic Acid
Transplant Drugs	Cyclosporine
Respiratory Drugs	Theophylline, Caffeine

Hair Tests

Levels of certain chemicals, drugs, and toxins can also be measured through analysis of hair samples from the mother and, under special conditions, the newborn. At the Motherisk Laboratory for Drug Exposure, for example, hair analysis is used to detect a broad range of drugs, and nicotine from environmental tobacco smoke.

Since maternal hair grows at approximately half an inch per month, tests can be done to several parts of a longer sample to determine concentrations in various sections of the hair. The validity of blood and urine tests depends on how long the drug stays in the blood or urine. Cocaine, for example, has a very short elimination half-life. That means that the drug is not likely to be detected for more than a few hours in blood and a few days in urine. In contrast, cocaine and other drugs can be detected in hair samples collected months after the drugs are consumed.

To date, no one can correlate the concentration of a drug in the hair with the exact amount and length of an individual's use of that drug. However, we can define mild, moderate, or high exposure.

FACT ✔ Passive or Systemic Exposures

Children's hair can be tested to detect passive or systemic exposure to smoke from crack, marijuana, or cigarettes. Newborn hair is tested to detect drug exposure before birth. The Motherisk Lab is also in the process of perfecting a method of hair analysis to detect alcohol exposure. For more information, contact Motherisk at www.motherisk.org or call (877) 327-4636 or (416) 813-8572.

Fetal Tests

Fetal tests and prenatal diagnosis may offer pregnant women and their partners the ability to make better informed choices during pregnancy. When the results of fetal tests are negative, they provide the basis for qualified reassurance (especially for those at high genetic risk). Fetal testing also offers the possibility of early diagnosis and treatment — either before or at birth. Prenatal diagnosis involves many different clinical and laboratory services. Ultrasound, amniocentesis, cordocentesis, and chorionic villus sampling are just four of the more common tests that you are likely to hear about during your pregnancy.

SAFETY/RISK ❖ Degree of Risk

If a major malformation is detected, the doctor managing your case will be able to estimate how serious it is. The decision whether to continue with the pregnancy or terminate it always resides with you and your family. The most important thing for you, whatever you decide, is to make an informed decision, based on full, up-to-date, evidence-based information. Talk to your health-care provider, ask to be referred to an expert, and ask questions.

Ultrasound

Ultrasound examination is a commonly used method to visualize the fetus. There is a wide range of quality in ultrasound examination, from crude analysis of the length of the fetus, to very detailed examination of the baby's external and internal organ.

When done after the first trimester of pregnancy (i.e., after more than 12 weeks of pregnancy), detailed ultrasound can see all external organs, including face and fingers. It also can detect some (but not all) problems in internal organs, such as the kidneys and heart. Ultrasound also evaluates the amniotic fluids, the water filling the uterus and surrounding the unborn baby.

There is no known risk to the unborn baby from ultrasound itself because the energy emitted during this procedure is minimal.

Amniocentesis

Amniocentesis is a procedure in which the doctor inserts a needle into the wall of the belly to reach the amniotic fluid, the liquid surrounding the fetus. This is done after freezing the skin, so the procedure itself should not be painful. This fluid contains fetal skin cells that allow analysis of the genetic material (chromosomes) of the baby and accurately identify genetic disorders such as Down Syndrome, Trisomy 18, and Fragile X Syndrome.

Analysis of the liquid itself can help identify neural tube defects by identifying high levels of alpha-fetoprotein, a protein produced in the baby and secreted into the amniotic fluid.

Amniocentesis is indicated only in limited cases. Women over the age of 35 have a higher rate of carrying babies with Down Syndrome, so the test is offered to them. It is also offered to women in whom blood tests or ultrasound suggest a risk for Down Syndrome.

Amniocentesis will also be offered to women who are known to have a genetic risk. That risk can be identified through this procedure. However, most women taking medications will not benefit from amniocentesis, as the test will not identify any risk factors, and the test itself, done at 16 weeks of pregnancy, carries a risk of around 1/1000 for miscarriage.

Reproduced by permission of the Prenatal Diagnosis and Medical Genetics Program, Mount Sinai Hospital, Toronto.

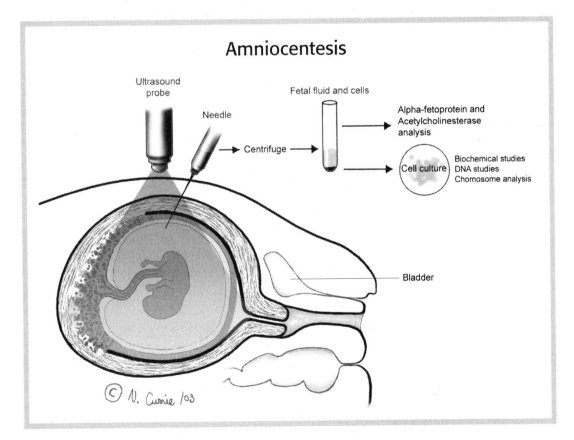

Amniocentesis

Cordocentesis

Cordocentesis or percutaneous umbilical blood sampling (PUBS) is a way of sampling blood from the umbilical cord. Cordocentesis is similar to amniocentesis except that it is used to collect fetal blood, rather than amniotic fluid. The procedure is performed by inserting a needle through the mother's belly and uterine wall. It is then guided by ultrasound into the umbilical artery and fetal blood is drawn.

This is not a routine test. It is offered in cases where ultrasound tests indicate a possible chromosomal problem. Fetal blood is also used to diagnose intrauterine infections, such as toxoplasmosis and rubella, and blood disorders, such as anemia and hemophilia. This procedure is also a way to administer medicines to the fetus. When called for, cordocentesis is conducted at a high-risk obstetric center. The procedure carries some risk of infection and miscarriage.

Chorionic Villus Sampling (CVS)

Chorionic villus sampling is done by inserting a small needle through the vagina into the placenta and taking a small sample of the placenta for examination. Because cells of the fetus create the placenta, this test allows genetic testing. Its main advantage over amniocentesis is that it can be performed earlier, at 10 to 12 weeks of pregnancy. Its main weakness is higher rate of miscarriage, up to 1%.

Reproduced by permission of the Prenatal Diagnosis and Medical Genetics Program, Mount Sinai Hospital, Toronto.

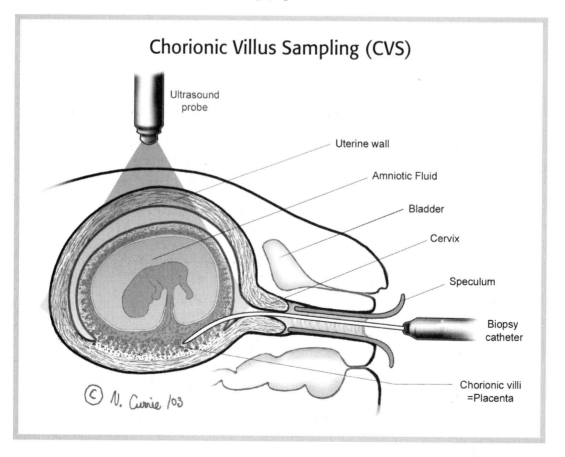

Chorionic Villus Sampling (CVS)

Ultrasound probe

Uterine wall

Amniotic Fluid

Bladder

Cervix

Speculum

Biopsy catheter

Chorionic villi =Placenta

© N. Currie /03

GUIDE TO SELECTED FETAL GENETIC DISORDERS
(Detected by Amniocentesis or Cordocentesis)

The following genetic disorders can be detected by amniocentesis or cordocentesis and analysis of fetal cells. This list can grow as new genetic discoveries are made that require additional testing.

Aceruloplasminemia
Achondroplasia
Adenosine Deaminase
Adrenoleukodystrophy
Alagille Syndrome
Alexander Disease
Alpha-thalassemia
Alpha1-antitrypsin Deficiency
Alkaptonuria
Alstrom Syndrome
Amyotrophic Lateral Sclerosis
Androgen Insensitivity Syndrome
Angelman Syndrome
Aniridia (Isolated)
Argininemia (Arginase Deficiency)
Arginosuccinicaciduria
Ataxia-Telangiectasia
Autosomal Recessive Congenital Ichthyosis

Bardet-Biedl Syndrome
Beckwith-Wiedemann Syndrome
Berardinelli-Seip Congenital Lipodystrophy
Beta-thalassemia
Biotinidase Deficiency

Canavan Disease
Carbamoylphosphate Synthetase I
   Deficiency (CPSI Deficiency)
Carney Complex
Cerebral Cavernous Malformation
Charcot-Marie-Tooth Disease
Childhood Ataxia with CNS Hypomyelination
Citrullinemia
Chromosal Aberrations (translocation,
   inversions, deletions, isochromosome,
   duplications, chromosome ring)
Cockayne Syndrome
Coffin-Lowry Syndrome
Congenital Adrenal Hyperplasia
Congenital Contractural Arachnodactyly

Congenital Myasthenic Syndrome
Craniosynostosis Syndromes
   (FGFR- Related)
Cri-Du-Chat Syndrome
Crouzon Syndrome
Cystic Fibrosis
Cystinuria
Cytomegalovirus Infection

Dentatorubral-Pallidoluysian Atrophy
DiGeorge Syndrome
Down Syndrome

Early Onset Familial Alzheimer Disease
Edwards Syndrome
Ehlers-Danlos Syndrome
Emery-Dreifuss Muscular Dystrophy
Epidermolysis Bullosa Simplex
Episodic Ataxia Type 2

Fabry Disease
Facioscapulohumeral Muscular Dystrophy
   (FSHD)
Familial Adenomatous Polyposis
Familial Char Syndrome
Familial Creutzfeldt-Jakob Disease
   (FCJD)
Familial Dysautonomia
Familial Hypercholesterolemia
Familial Hyperinsulinism
Familial Mediterranean Fever
Fanconi Anemia
Fragile X Syndrome
Friedreich Ataxia

Galactosemia
Gaucher Disease
Giant Axonal Neuropathy
GM1-gangliosidosis
Greig Cephalopolysyndactyly Syndrome

Hemophilia A and B
Hereditary Hemorrhagic Telangiectasia
Hereditary Multiple Exostoses
Hereditary Neuropathy (with liability to
   pressure palsies)
Hereditary Sensory Neuropathy
   Type I
Hereditary Spastic Paraplegia
Hermansky-Pudlak Syndrome
Hippel-Lindau Syndrome
Homocystinuria
Hunter Syndrome
Huntington Disease
Hurler Syndrome
Hutchinson-Gilford Progeria Syndrome
Hypokalemic Periodic Paralysis

Incontinentia Pigmenti

Jervell and Lange-Nielsen Syndrome
Juvenile Polyposis Syndrome

Klinefelter Syndrome
Krabbe Disease

Lesch-Nyhan Syndrome
Li Fraumeni Syndrome
Limb-Girdle Muscular Dystrophy
Lowe Syndrome
L/S (ratio for lung maturity)

Malignant Hyperthermia Susceptibility
Maple Syrup Urine Disease
Marfan Syndrome
Medium-Chain Acyl-Coenzyme A
   Dehydrogenase Deficiency
Megalencephalic Leukoencephalopathy
   with Subcortical Cysts
Methylmalonic Acidemia
Morquio Disease
Multiminicore Disease
Multiple Endocrine Neoplasia
   Type 2
Multiple Epiphyseal Dysplasia
Muscular Dystrophy
Myotonic Dystrophy
Myoclonus-Dystonia

N-acetyl Glutamate Synthetase Deficiency
   (NAGS Deficiency)
Nail-Patella Syndrome
Nemaline Myopathy
Nephrogenic Diabetes Insipidus
Neural Tube Defect (NTD)
Neurofibromatosis
Neuronal Ceroid-Lipofuscinoses
Nevoid Basal Cell Carcinoma Syndrome
Niemann-Pick Disease
Nijmegen Breakage Syndrome
Nonsyndromic Hearing Loss and Deafness,
   DFNA3, DFNB1
Noonan Syndrome
Norrie Disease

Oculocutaneous Albinism
   Type 1 and 2
Ornithine Transcarbamylase Deficiency
   (OTC Deficiency)
Osteogenesis Imperfecta

Pallister-Hall Syndrome
Pantothenate Kinase-Associated
   Neurodegeneration
Patau Syndrome
Pelizaeus-Merzbacher Disease
Pendred Syndrome
Peroxisome Biogenesis Disorders
Peutz-Jeghers Syndrome
Phenylketonuria
Polycystic Kidney Disease
Prader-Willi Syndrome
Primary Hyperoxaluria
   Type 1
Progressive Familial Intrahepatic
   Cholestasis 1 and 2
PROP 1-Related Combined Pituitary
   Hormone Deficiency (CPHD)
PTEN Hamartoma Tumor Syndrome

Retinoblastoma
Rett Syndrome
Rhizomelic Chondrodysplasia Punctata
   Type I
Romano-Ward Syndrome
Rubinstein-Taybi Syndrome

Saethre-Chotzen Syndrome
Sanfilippo Syndrome
Sialuria
Sickle Cell Anemia
Smith-Lemli-Opitz Syndrome
Smith-Magenis Syndrome
SOST-Related Sclerosing Bone Dysplasias
SPG4 Spinal Muscular Atrophy
Spinal and Bulbar Muscular Atrophy
Spinal Muscular Atrophy
Spinocerebellar Ataxia
Stickler Syndrome

Tay Sachs Disease
Thoracic Aortic Aneurysms
    and Aortic Dissection

Transthyretin Amyloidosis
Tuberous Sclerosis Complex

Waardenburg Syndrome Type 1
Werner Syndrome
Williams Syndrome
Wilson's Disease
Wolf-Hirschhorn Syndrome

Xeroderma Pigmentosa
X-Linked Juvenile Retinoschisis
X-Linked Myotubular Myopathy
X-Linked Severe Combined Immunodeficiency
XX Male Syndrome

Zellweger Syndrome Spectrum

Testing the Newborn

In some cases of exposure to medications in pregnancy, it is equally important to monitor the baby after birth. Your doctor will want to ensure that your baby is responding appropriately to the child's environment, achieving age appropriate milestones, and developing normally.

Withdrawal Syndrome

Some drugs can produce a withdrawal or 'discontinuation' syndrome in babies, as in adults. When a pregnant woman uses benzodiazepine (such as Valium or Xanax), opioids or narcotics (such as codeine or morphine) alcohol, SSRIs, or barbiturates, the newborn baby may crave the drug and display irritability, inconsolable crying, diarrhea, vomiting, tremors, dehydration, and even seizures.

If you are taking any of these medications in late pregnancy, it is important for you to report this to the health-care professionals attending the birth, so that appropriate monitoring and treatment, if needed, are initiated.

If treated appropriately, a withdrawal syndrome by itself is not a sign of bad things to come in the long-term health of the child. Though the affected newborn may need special care and treatment at first, after that initial period the child may continue to develop normally. The child's mother and healthcare provider will want to monitor the child to see that normal milestones of growth and development are met.

RESOURCES

The medical literature includes many sources of information on genetic disorders and prenatal diagnosis. The following list is just a small sample of what you can find if you wish to read more on this topic. Another helpful resource is the March of Dimes website at www.modimes.org.

Koren G, ed. Maternal-Fetal Toxicology. A Clinician's Guide. 3rd ed. New York: Marcel Dekker, 2001.

Harper PS. Practical Genetic Counselling. 5th ed. Boston: Butterworth Heinemann, 1998.

Hook EB. Rates of chromosome abnormalities at different maternal ages. Obstetrics and Gynecology 1981;58:282-85.

Brock DJH, Rodeck CH, Ferguson-Smith MA, eds. Prenatal Diagnosis and Screening. New York: Churchill Livingston, 1992.

Testing Women for HIV

Q My doctor talked to me about screening for HIV, but I don't think I have a risk. Should I bother?

A Many HIV-infected pregnant women are unaware of their HIV status, and their infection goes undetected until either they or their children develop symptoms. Though you may not feel you are at risk, it is currently recommended that all pregnant women be offered an HIV screening test as part of their prenatal care. The HIV test is performed only after counseling and obtaining informed consent.

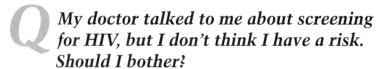

FACT ✔ **Transmission Rates**

HIV can be transmitted from mother to child during gestation and delivery or through breast milk. The rate of transmission of HIV from mother to child during pregnancy without intervention ranges between 15% and 40%; the rate with optimal antiretroviral (ARV) management is 1% to 3%, and in some studies, even zero.

In-Depth

Perinatal transmission of Human Immunodeficiency Virus (HIV) — the transmission of the disease from mother to baby any time between the 28th week of pregnancy through 28 days following birth — is the main cause of HIV infection and subsequent death in North American children today.

In the United States, about 7,000 HIV-positive women become pregnant each year and 1,000 to 2,000 of their babies are born HIV-positive. Several studies of women of childbearing age lead us to estimate that about 120 infants are born to HIV-positive women each year.

Risk factors for HIV include illicit drug use, having multiple sexual partners, and having a male partner with multiple sexual partners. Women have made up an increasing proportion of those with newly diagnosed HIV infections over the last few years and now account for about 20% of newly diagnosed cases. Most of these women are of childbearing age.

The rate of mother-to-infant transmission of HIV type 1 infection in the absence of therapeutic intervention is between 15% and 40%. Between 25% and 50% of all children with perinatally acquired HIV infection develop clinical AIDS within their first year, and 80% develop it within 3 to 5 years.

Testing for HIV during pregnancy provides an important opportunity for starting antiretroviral (ARV) treatment if necessary. Therapy for the mother reduces the risk of HIV transmission to her child.

While zidovudine monotherapy was initially the most frequently prescribed treatment, combination therapy is now more common.

RESOURCES

HIV Healthline: To enable HIV-positive women to make informed decisions regarding ARV treatment, Motherisk, in collaboration with the Pediatric HIV Program at The Hospital for Sick Children in Toronto, established the HIV Healthline: (888) 246-5840. Our goal is to provide up-to-date information regarding the effectiveness and safety of ARV drugs. The HIV Healthline can provide information to HIV-positive women about counseling and follow-up.

CHAPTER FIVE

Morning Sickness

I cried when I read an announcement about your NVP (morning sickness) helpline. I suffered with severe morning sickness twice. I was lucky and now have two beautiful, healthy daughters. I still look at my girls for signs of abnormalities due to being so ill... I wish I had known then where to turn...

— *Motherisk Caller*

Nausea and vomiting of pregnancy (NVP), more commonly known as morning sickness, can turn the most welcome pregnancy into a desperate and even life-threatening condition. All too often, morning sickness goes untreated because physicians, pharmacists, and other health-care professionals are unsure of the safety or risk of available treatments. A 1997 Motherisk study of the consequences of morning sickness found that many women suffer needlessly from this condition and that misinformation and medical mismanagement of morning sickness has had disastrous effects.

Causes of Morning Sickness

The exact cause of morning sickness is not known. While many researchers believe it has to do with hormone changes in pregnancy, no one yet has identified a specific hormone that causes these symptoms. Researchers have studied a variety of mechanisms involving thyroid, parathyroid, and hepatic dysfunction; gestational hormone alteration; blunting of autonomic nervous system function with decreased gastric emptying; alterations in carbohydrate metabolism; and nutritional deficiencies. Evidence for these mechanisms is contradictory or preliminary. Psychological factors, such as depression, anxiety, and interpersonal conflicts, have also been observed, but whether symptoms come before psychological disturbance or vice versa is not clear.

FACT ✔ **Insidious Side-Effect**

An insidious side-effect of NVP is the harm caused by the unfounded belief that severe morning sickness reflects a conscious or subconscious rejection of the pregnancy. The 1997 Motherisk study utterly rejected this view, showing that women are ready to endure immense suffering before giving up a wanted pregnancy. The study also uncovered the fact that many women were not offered approved medication because their doctors mistakenly believed that it was a harmful teratogen.

Prevalence of NVP

Nausea and vomiting during pregnancy afflicts up to 80% of pregnant women to some degree; 50% have nausea and vomiting; 30% have nausea only. Although usually limited to the first 7 to 12 weeks of gestation, 9% of patients continue to have symptoms beyond 20 weeks.

The suffering is real. In mild forms, the nausea and vomiting of pregnancy adversely affect the quality of life of the pregnant woman and her family. Those with severe symptoms may experience nausea every 30 minutes and may vomit as many as 15 times a day. The toll on the woman, as well as on her partner and family, is immense. The 1997 Motherisk study of morning sickness showed that some women may even terminate otherwise wanted pregnancies due to extreme morning sickness.

Less than 1% of pregnant women develop hyperemesis gravidarum (HG), which is characterized by intractable nausea and vomiting; severe interference with daily life; and medical complications, such as dehydration, metabolic abnormalities, and weight loss, leading to hospital admission. The severity and duration of NVP during previous pregnancies is a poor indicator of symptoms during subsequent pregnancies.

Coping Strategies

Although we don't really understand the cause of NVP and HG, researchers and clinicians fortunately know significantly more about ways to control NVP. Pregnant women have found varying levels of relief by snacking instead of dining, avoiding certain foods and smells, using acupressure techniques such as wrist 'sea bands', ingesting ginger, and trying hypnotherapy. Another strategy is to avoid the intake of liquids while you are ingesting food. If you need to quench your thirst, do it before or after you have eaten something — not at the same time.

The effectiveness of these and other strategies have not been scientifically proven, though they seem to help many women. For more anecdotal accounts of what may or may not work, visit the Motherisk NVP Forum at www.motherisk.org/forum and read about what others have tried under "Coping." Here are just a few samples.

Questions from the Motherisk NVP Forum

Q I'm 26 years old and have two wonderful children, but being pregnant with them wasn't easy. My greatest problem was morning sickness. In fact, it was so bad that I had trouble functioning. I ended up losing weight, quitting work, and couldn't look after my home and family. I'd love to have another child, but I don't know if I could face the misery of morning sickness again. Is there something I can do to avoid it?

A No two pregnancies are alike. With any luck, morning sickness won't be the debilitating problem it was the first two times around. Even if you expect the worst, there is safe and effective medication for morning sickness. Our Motherisk NVP Helpline counselors (800-436-8477) are also available to suggest helpful strategies to cope with your symptoms, and to recommend ways for you to ensure that you are using the medication in the right dose and at the right time.

Q I have had severe nausea for more than 2 weeks now and have lost weight and am more than 2 months pregnant. I can't stand soup and Gatorade anymore and don't know what else I can try to eat. Toast, cheese, crackers with peanut butter are all bad (cause me to throw up). One thing I ate that was okay was oven-baked herb salmon, but I have no idea why and can't eat it everyday. I am at a loss as to how to try to eat because I'm getting weak and have lost quite a bit of weight. Can you help?

> **SAFETY/RISK**
>
> **Safe Treatment**
> If NVP remains a major issue, not relieved by any of these methods, you should discuss it with your doctor. Safe, approved treatment is available.

A Women suffering from NVP may have difficulty eating during their first trimester. What's more, people have different likes and dislikes when it comes to food.

We suggest that you eat a very small amount of any food or snack frequently (hourly, more or less). Continue this frequent "nibbling" (not more than a bite or two) during the night just to keep something in your stomach at all times. Avoid cooking. Liquids (a few sips) should be consumed half an hour before or after you eat — not while you are eating.

For women who are unable to eat in the manner described above, we suggest a can of food supplement (such as Boost or Ensure) in a blender, diluted with ice cubes. This can be eaten like a slushy — one small spoonful at a time.

In Canada, Diclectin (vitamin B-6 and doxylamine succinate) is the only approved medication for NVP. There's lots of information on the Motherisk website about Diclectin. A treatment algorithm is also included in the February 2002 Motherisk Update at www.motherisk.org/updates/index.php?id=348>.

Q I'm 30 years old and pregnant. I have asthma and am taking prednisone under my doctor's supervision. Whenever my doctor decreases my prednisone dose, my nausea increases tremendously, even though I am taking two tablets of Diclectin daily. I am already at 26 weeks gestation, and I really do not want to continue the prednisone beyond what is needed for my asthma, but two attempts to taper prednisone off has failed because of unbearable nausea. Do you have any advice?

*A*Several controlled trials show the efficacy of prednisone for nausea and vomiting of pregnancy (NVP), but your case is fascinating in proving the point. Your doctor should try to decrease the prednisone while increasing doxylamine and pyridoxine to its recommended dose of two tablets before sleep, one in the morning, and one in the afternoon. Many physicians now increase the dose of Diclectin to even 6 or 8 tablets. Your doctor should also consider several key points that were established in the Canadian Consensus on the management of NVP.

MANAGING MORNING SICKNESS (NVP)

The Consensus

The medical establishment can pride itself on several initiatives aimed at improving management of women suffering from NVP. Many of these initiatives have helped bring to an end the typical trivialization of this medical condition.

In 1997, The Society for Obstetricians and Gynaecologists of Canada produced an effective pamphlet on management of NVP. The same year, Motherisk initiated the NVP Helpline to counsel and support women and health professionals in managing this condition.

In 1998, the Canadian Consensus on NVP was developed by a national group of family physicians, obstetricians, internists, clinical pharmacologists, nurses, and dietitians. What follow are several key points in management of NVP as they appear in the Consensus. These points are supported by findings from Motherisk research.

Patient-Centered

Different women have different needs. A certain number of vomiting incidents daily, for example, could be well tolerated by one woman but disastrous to another. Nausea itself can be very debilitating.

For example, among 256 women who called the Motherisk NVP Helpline about their main concerns regarding NVP, 140 (53.8%) identified nausea as most bothersome, while only 19 (7.3%) mentioned vomiting, and 97 (37.3%) were concerned about both.

Motherisk research has discovered high rates of psychosocial suffering among women with NVP, including depression, rage, and a sense of isolation. Time lost from work or serious adverse effects on family life can be devastating. Women should not be told "it is all in their heads." Many health professionals still do that, despite there being no proof. Nothing is more frustrating to a woman than telling her that NVP is due to her "rejection of the pregnancy."

Associated Conditions

Multiple pregnancies, molar pregnancies (an abnormality of the placenta), and hydramnios (a condition during pregnancy characterized by too much amniotic fluid) increase the likelihood and severity of NVP. Other conditions with similar effects include drug toxicity, diabetes, central nervous system lesions, ketoacidosis, hyperthyroidism, and vestibular disorders.

Diagnoses other than Nausea and Vomiting of Pregnancy

Among the thousands of women in the first trimester of pregnancy in Canada every year, some could have other conditions that manifest as nausea and vomiting, but are not pregnancy-related morning sickness. Some of these conditions include:

Gastrointestinal Diseases
- Peptic Disorders
- Appendicitis
- Viral Gastroenteritis
- Irritable Bowel Disorder
- Bowel Obstruction
- Pancreatitis

Liver Diseases
- Hepatitis

Genitourinary Tract Diseases
- Urinary Tract Infection
- Ovarian Torsion
- Fibroid Degeneration
- Uremia

Effective Doses of Safe Drugs

When doctors prescribe medication for your NVP, they should be sure to prescribe an effective dose. Subtherapeutic (less than therapeutic) doses of prescribed drugs are not helpful. Two tablets of doxylamine and pyridoxine in the evening help morning symptoms of NVP for most women because the drug is delayed-release, but this regimen might not address symptoms at noon or in the evening. An additional morning tablet will help most patients around noon and during the afternoon, and, when needed, a tablet at noon will help in the evening.

Medications for Treating NVP

Bendectin and Diclectin

The story of Diclectin and its American predecessor, Bendectin, is a fascinating illustration of the gap that often exists between the perception of risk and evidence-based proof of safety.

Bendectin

During the 1950s and '60s, Bendectin, a combination of an antihistamine (doxylamine) and pyridoxine, was the most widely used medication in the United States for NVP. In the 1970s, the drug's manufacturer was sued repeatedly in American courts, based on unproven claims that Bendectin was teratogenic. Though not a teratogen, Bendectin became a costly "litogen" (subject of repeated litigation), and was eventually removed from the market by a manufacturer that presumably had had enough of the legal wrangling.

Bendectin was withdrawn despite a substantial body of evidence that showed that the rate of major malformations among the children of women who used Bendectin did not differ from the rate in the general population. What's more, though

RESOURCES
Physicians and patients alike are welcome to call the Motherisk NVP Helpline at (800) 436-8477. Many coping strategies are listed in the questions and answers posted on the Motherisk NVP Forum at www.motherisk.org /forum/.

Bendectin was used by up to 40% of pregnant women at one time, its removal from the market was not accompanied by a decrease in the rate of any specific malformations — as would be expected after the removal of a truly teratogenic drug. Instead, what did occur was a three-fold increase in the rates of hospitalization of women for management of severe forms of NVP.

Diclectin

The situation in Canada is not nearly so troubling where the drug is marketed under the name Diclectin. Studied in about 200,000 pregnant women and found to be safe, Diclectin is the only drug specifically labeled and approved for use in NVP. Diclectin is a delayed-release tablet and, as such, is not useful for acute management of NVP and HG. But used in the right dose and with the right timing, Diclectin can provide significant relief. A Motherisk study showed that in women who had previously very severe morning sickness, pre-emptive therapy (i.e., starting the medication with the very first symptoms) prevented in many cases the severe course from recurring. The antihistamine component of Diclectin, like other antihistamines, sometimes causes drowsiness and anticholinergic signs and symptoms.

Other Medications

Other medications, such as dimenhydrinate (Gravol), hydroxyzine (Atarax), meclizine (Antivert), and phenothiazines such as chlorpromazine (Largactil), prochlorperazine (Stemetil), and promethazine (Phenergan), also have not demonstrated teratogenicity, although many fewer pregnant patients have been studied with these drugs. These medications are also available in formulations that provide acute relief, especially for women with HG, though they may be sedating. Phenothiazines may have other effects, as well.

Corticosteroids have not demonstrated serious teratogenic potential in humans. Data on human safety are limited but reassuring for cisapride (Prepulsid), metoclopramide (e.g., Maxeran), and ondansetron (Zofran). There are no human safety data for domperidone (e.g., Motilium).

Efficacy is as important as safety, but evidence-based information is relatively scant. Only doxylamine and pyridoxine were shown to be effective compared with placebo in more than 2,000 patients. Small, randomized placebo-controlled trials have shown that all of the following are effective for treating or preventing NVP and HG: other histamine (H_1) antagonists (e.g., hydroxyzine, meclizine), phenothiazines (e.g., promethazine), and P6 acupressure. Pyridoxine alone might be effective, at least when contained within a multivitamin. Case series have suggested that corticosteroids, prokinetic agents (metoclopramide, cisapride), ondansetron, and electrical vestibular stimulation are therapeutic.

In Canada, your doctor is most likely to prescribe an optimal dose of Diclectin (e.g., two tablets before bed, one in the morning, and one mid-afternoon). Since Diclectin is not available outside of Canada, physicians may prescribe similar combinations of doxylamine and pyridoxine, though only Diclectin is available in time-release formulation.

MEDICATIONS EFFECTIVE FOR MORNING SICKNESS

Research studies have shown these medications are effective for morning sickness, without significant risk to fetal safety.

Chemical Name	Brand Name
Doxylamine & Pyridoxine	Diclectin (a delayed-release medication that combines these two drugs). Diclectin is presently available in Canada only.
Dimenhydrinate	Gravol
Promethazine	Phenergan
Chlorpromazine	Largactil
Prochlorperazine	Stemetil
Metoclopramide	Reglan; Maxeran
Ondansetron	Zofran

RESOURCES

You can read more about morning sickness (NVP) on the Motherisk website at www.motherisk.org. Our on-line resources include:

Nausea and vomiting of pregnancy: Evidence-based treatment algorithm. Full text available in the February 2002 Motherisk Update posted on the Motherisk website under "Newsletters and Updates - Archives."

Nausea and Vomiting of Pregnancy: State of the Art 2000. Full text available at www.nvp-volumes.org

CHAPTER SIX

Prescription Drugs

I was so pleased, as the father of an expecting child (my wife is having a baby!), to find your site. The information you provide is excellent and in a world were so many questions need to be answered, this website delivers (literally!). Thank you so much for all the hard work and dedication you have put into this website — it will carry me into the next 6 months before my child is born into this very interesting world!

— Signed: A Father-to-Be

Pregnancy, whether planned or a pleasant surprise, brings with it important concerns about prescription and over-the-counter drugs. Not every medication poses a risk to your unborn baby. However, some do. Talk to your doctor. Discuss the relative risks and benefits of any prescribed drug therapy and do *not* take over-the-counter drugs, herbal remedies, or vitamin and mineral supplements without first consulting your physician.

If you are already pregnant, Motherisk's published research can help you and your doctor make informed decisions about possible drug therapy. Since 1985, Motherisk has reviewed data from around the world, conducting controlled, prospective studies to determine the potential risks of therapeutic drugs during pregnancy. It is now clear that there are many drugs that are unlikely to pose a risk to your unborn child.

Understanding Drug Safety

Before proceeding to the list of prescription medications below (medications that you can only get with a doctor's note), we need to recall the issue discussed in the Introduction called

RISK GRADES

At Motherisk, we have established a system for grading the risk of prescription and over-the-counter drugs in pregnancy, ranging from 'Safe' to 'Unsafe'. This does not mean that everything that is not deemed 'Safe' is 'Unsafe' and must be avoided during pregnancy. There are *degrees of safety* that should be considered, especially if the medication is important for the health and well-being of the mother. These degrees of safety are vital to balancing the benefit and the risk of various medications.

Safe

Safe means that a convincing and authoritative body of scientific evidence, accumulated over time, through sound scientific research, shows no adverse effects on the fetus.

Probably Safe

Probably Safe means that there is no evidence the drug is dangerous to the fetus and that the information showing it to be safe is rather large. Here, the benefit/risk assessment will be weighted, in most cases, in favor of using the medication.

Possibly Safe

Possibly Safe means that there is no evidence that the drug is dangerous for the fetus, but the information showing it to be safe is limited. By 'limited' we mean that only a few studies have been published in the medical literature, or the studies that are available do not meet all of the rigorous standards of critical scientific appraisal.

Unsafe

Unsafe means that there is evidence to show that the medication may cause harmful effects during pregnancy or during a particular trimester of pregnancy. This does not mean that the harm is certain to happen in each and every case of exposure, but there is enough risk of harm to justify careful use or avoidance in pregnancy.

Unknown or Unclear

Unknown or *Unclear* means that there is simply not enough reliable information for us to be able to determine safety or risk in pregnancy. This may change over time as evidence-based research uncovers more information about the effects of these drugs.

"Risk Assessment and Management." Some drugs pose a greater risk than others, but there are many options for rational drug therapy in pregnancy.

Though drug manufacturers must establish the safety and effectiveness of their medications before the drugs are approved by the government regulatory agencies for sale, clinical trials are rarely conducted on pregnant women. Drug safety in pregnancy is generally determined after the drug appears on the market, through a process called *post-marketing surveillance*. It makes sense, then, that the longer a drug has been on the market, the more evidence we will collect about its effects. The more reports gathered from pregnant women on any given medication, the more confident we can be about statements regarding its likely effect in pregnancy. When we talk about the risk or safety of any given medication, we are really talking about the quantity and quality of the evidence collected to-date.

FREQUENTLY ASKED QUESTIONS

Accutane

Q: I took Accutane and it was very effective in clearing up my acne. I was told I should not conceive while taking Accutane and so I have been taking birth control pills. To my surprise, I now find that I am 7 weeks pregnant. According to my calculations, it seems I took several tablets of Accutane unknowingly within the first 4 weeks of pregnancy. Am I in the 'Safe Zone' because of the small dose?

A: Unfortunately not. Malformations have been described even after fetal exposure to low doses (a few tablets) of Accutane.

Ampicillin, Nitrofurantoin & Other Antibiotics

Q: I am 5 weeks pregnant and have urinary urgency. My doctor did a urine test and says I have an infection. I am afraid to take antibiotics for the infection. What should I do?

A: First-line antibiotics for urinary infection do not pose a risk to the baby. This includes ampicillin and nitrofurantoin. Untreated urinary tract infection is associated with increased risk for prematurity and perinatal complications.

Depakene for Epilepsy

Q: I am treated with Depakene for epilepsy and really doing well. Now we want to start a family, but I don't know what to do about treating my condition during pregnancy. On the one hand, my doctor tells me that Depakene causes spina bifida in some babies and I am afraid to continue on the drug. On the other hand, I am very worried about discontinuing my medication because the one time I tried to stop last year I had several seizures. Do you have any advice?

A: You and your baby will need to be carefully monitored by your doctor. The first thing your physician will recommend is that you take a high dose of folic acid (4 mg/day). Your doctor should also send you for detailed level 2 ultrasound and blood tests for alpha-fetoproteins. These can rule out neural tube defects such as spina bifida. Depakene may also cause other malformations – of the heart, for example.

Warfarin Use

Q I have been taking warfarin for some time for treatment of deep vein thrombosis. I just found out that I am pregnant and I don't know what to do. Is there evidence that warfarin use during pregnancy is associated with fetal risk?

A If possible, warfarin therapy should be avoided during pregnancy. If warfarin therapy is essential, it should be avoided at least during the first trimester (because of teratogenicity) and from about 2 to 4 weeks before delivery to reduce risk of bleeding complications. Unfractionated heparin or low-molecular weight heparin could be substituted *when appropriate* because these agents do not cross the placenta and are considered the anticoagulant drugs of choice during pregnancy.

FACT ✓ Fetal Warfarin Syndrome

Several reports have indicated that using warfarin between 6 and 12 weeks of pregnancy is associated with Fetal Warfarin Syndrome, which is most commonly manifested by skeletal abnormalities and respiratory distress. Also, use of warfarin during the second and third trimesters has been associated sporadically with central nervous system abnormalities, including mental retardation, microcephaly, optic atrophy, and blindness.

In-Depth

Warfarin (Coumadin) is an oral anticoagulant (inhibits blood clot formation). Rats given very high doses (100 mg/kg) of warfarin have had offspring with abnormal development of the midface and skeleton.

Several case series and case reports of human use of warfarin during pregnancy have been published. These reports (which range in size from one to 418 subjects) show a clear association between warfarin therapy and embryo development disorder. The exact risk of fetal damage from warfarin therapy during pregnancy is difficult to determine because most of the available studies are small and anecdotal.

Other fetal abnormalities reported with maternal warfarin use include absent or nonfunctioning kidneys, anal dysplasia, deafness, seizures, Dandy-Walker syndrome, and other effects on the brain. Use of warfarin throughout pregnancy has been associated with bleeding complications, premature births, spontaneous abortions, stillbirths, and death.

The literature suggests a strong association between maternal warfarin use and fetal adverse effects. The most recent review recommends that women receiving long-term oral anticoagulation have warfarin replaced with unfractionated or low-molecular weight heparin when they become pregnant.

However, there have been case reports of unfractionated heparin being associated with adverse pregnancy outcomes, such as fetal loss and maternal bleeding, hemorrhage, and osteoporosis. Needless to say, the women in these studies were often sick, and their complications could have been caused by an underlying illness. A study of 108 women who received low-molecular weight heparin showed no increase above baseline for fetal deaths or malformations. Still, it is important that the risk and benefits of these alternatives to warfarin be considered and discussed with your doctor.

Anti-Anxiety Drugs (Benzodiazepines)

Q *I suffer from anxiety and was using lorazepam, a benzodiazepine drug, to treat it. The lorazepam worked well for me. That was before I found out that I was pregnant. As soon as I realized I was pregnant, I stopped taking the medication. Now I am worried about the potential effect on my baby. Are benzodiazepines safe during pregnancy? What should I do if I need anti-anxiety treatment during the rest of my pregnancy?*

A The study of benzodiazepines (BZDs) is an interesting illustration of what researchers can do when they are presented with studies that produce different results. In the case of BZDs, data from *case-control studies* show a slightly increased risk of oral cleft in exposed fetuses. In contrast, evidence gathered from *cohort studies* does not identify a notable association between the use of BZDs and increased risk of major malformations — including oral cleft. So Motherisk researchers decided to conduct a *meta-analysis* to try to arrive at some conclusions about the use of BZDs; the research methodology and findings are described below.

In-Depth

Benzodiazepines (BZDs) are commonly used for anxiety and insomnia, even by pregnant women. Because about one half of all pregnancies are unplanned, many women could inadvertently expose fetuses to BZDs during the first trimester.

The use of BZDs during pregnancy has been associated with teratogenic effects, such as facial cleft and skeletal anomalies, in some animal studies but not in others. Early human case-control studies suggested that maternal exposure to BZDs increases the risk of fetal cleft lip and cleft palate. Other reports have implicated BZDs in other major malformations, abnormal neurodevelopment, and a congenital benzodiazepine syndrome similar to Fetal Alcohol Syndrome.

Unfortunately, these studies were not designed to control for outside factors that could have influenced the results. Several prospective cohort studies involving hundreds of women using BZDs during pregnancy and an equal number of controls failed to show increased risk of malformations after BZD use during the first trimester.

These contradictory results have led to considerable controversy surrounding the use of BZDs during pregnancy. Nevertheless, it seemed clear that, even if it existed, the risk of malformations in newborns exposed to BZDs during the first trimester was marginal. To investigate this issue, Motherisk conducted a meta-analysis of all data on exposure to BZDs during the first trimester.

SAFETY/RISK

Level 2 Ultrasonography

BZDs do not seem to be major human teratogens; however, because some cases of cleft lip can be visualized by fetal ultrasound, level 2 ultrasonography should be used to rule out this malformation. Using BZDs late in pregnancy may cause withdrawal syndrome in newborns.

Meta-Analysis

As in the case of BZD use during pregnancy, researchers are often presented with studies that produce different results. The problem is how to analyze the data to arrive at an overall conclusion concerning a drug's risk or safety. A mathematical method has been developed to arrive at a single overall value that describes the relationship between a drug and a particular outcome or effect. That method is called meta-analysis and involves the statistical combination of research from independent studies. It has become increasingly popular among researchers as a way of summarizing the results of studies found in the medical literature.

Motherisk's Meta-Analysis of BZD

Motherisk considered 13 studies that examined major malformations, 11 that examined oral cleft alone, and three that examined other specific malformations. Various BZDs were used or prescribed, although nearly half of the studies examined use of chlordiazepoxide or diazepam only.

Data from *cohort studies* (studies that compared a group of exposed subjects with a group of nonexposed subjects) showed no significant association between BZDs during the first trimester and either major malformations or oral cleft alone. However, data from *case-control studies* (studies that began with a particular outcome and searched the records for evidence of exposure to the drug) showed a small but significant increased risk for these outcomes.

Motherisk's BZD meta-analysis helped to illustrate the advantages and disadvantages of the cohort vs. case-control studies of BZDs and supported researchers' determination that BZDs do not seem to be major human teratogens. Because some cases of cleft lip can be visualized by fetal ultrasound, level 2 ultrasonography should still be used to rule out this malformation.

Acid-Suppressing Drugs

Q *I suffer from a severe form of gastroesophageal reflux and regurgitation. I have tried to manage my condition with antacids, but they don't work. Now that I'm pregnant, I worry about taking acid-suppressing drugs. What can you tell me about their safety in pregnancy?*

*A*cid-suppressing drugs, mainly H_2-blockers and omeprazole, do not appear to cause measurable teratogenic risk in humans. Given the much wider experience with ranitidine than with omeprazole, however, ranitidine should remain the drug of choice at present. A growing body of information about omeprazole and initial reassuring results could mean that this drug will be added to first-line therapy in the future.

In-Depth

Gastroesophageal reflux is the backflow of stomach contents (typically acid) into the esophagus. One of the main symptoms is heartburn, a burning sensation that radiates up to the neck, often after lying down. Heartburn affects 30% to 50% of all pregnant women and tends to get worse as pregnancy advances. Upper abdominal pain, regurgitation, and heartburn can be severe. Some women restrict their meals to once daily due to severe symptoms after eating; others are forced to sleep upright all night.

The main goal of treatment is to relieve symptoms. Effective acid-suppressing drugs are available now for treating peptic and gastric ulcer, reflux esophagitis, and Zollinger-Ellison Syndrome. Data on the safety of acid-suppressing drugs during human pregnancy are, however, scarce. To address this issue, we searched the medical literature published up to 1997 with omeprazole and H_2-antagonists as key words.

Safety of H_2-blocker Use in Early Pregnancy

All H_2-blockers cross the human placenta. Animal reproductive toxicology studies, however, failed to show that any of the H_2-blockers were teratogenic. As for the results of human exposure, neither postmarketing surveillance conducted by North American drug manufacturers nor anecdotal reports of cimetidine or ranitidine exposure during the first trimester have reported evidence of teratogenicity. The same is true of record linkage studies and in the Michigan Medicaid Surveillance Study (conducted from 1985 to 1992).

In a prospective study on the topic, 178 (77.4%) of a possible 230 women who called the Motherisk Program about gestational H_2-blocker use were recruited. Their pregnancy outcomes were compared with those of 178 controls matched for age, smoking, and heavy alcohol consumption. Most patients ingested ranitidine; others took cimetidine, famotidine, and nizatidine. The primary indication was heartburn (41%), followed by peptic ulcer

---

FACT ✔

H_2-blocker Exposure

No evidence indicates that H_2-blocker exposure during the first trimester is associated with increased risk of major malformations above the baseline risk of 1% to 5% in all pregnancies.

disease (30%), epigastric pain (17%), and other conditions (12%). No increase in major malformations was found following first-trimester exposure to H_2-blockers: three of 142 (2.1%) H_2-blocker users had infants with major malformations compared with five of 143 (3.5%) controls.

Safety of H_2-blocker Use Later in Pregnancy

There is little information on the effect on fetal or neonatal outcomes of taking H_2-blockers later in pregnancy. So far, all we have to go on are the results of the prospective Motherisk study described briefly above. In that study, no aspects of pregnancy outcome (including prematurity and low birth weight) or newborn health differed between H_2-blocker users and controls, even when outcomes of only the 22% of newborns exposed to H_2-blockers at delivery were analyzed. Nor did the incidence of jaundice differ between groups of users versus controls. More studies are needed, however, to confirm the safety of these agents during late pregnancy.

SAFETY/RISK ❖ Lifestyle Modifications

Patients with uncomplicated reflux may want to consider lifestyle modifications first. Although these measures have not been *proven* effective by clinical trials, they are safe, inexpensive, and appear to be effective for many patients. Such measures include elevating the head of the bed, avoiding bedtime snacks or late meals, choosing low-fat foods, quitting smoking, and controlling symptoms with antacids or alginic acid.

Safety of Omeprazole

Omeprazole has been shown to be very efficient for treating duodenal and gastric ulcer and is the drug of choice for reflux esophagitis. Although it crosses the placenta, animal studies failed to show drug-induced teratogenicity following doses 250 to 500 times the recommended dose for humans. Human data are scarce and consist of a few published case reports and spontaneous reports to the manufacturers. In these reports, there was no consistency in type of abnormality reported or stage of pregnancy when the mother was exposed to omeprazole.

Hypertension Medications

Q *I have had hypertension (high blood pressure) for 6 years. Now I am planning to get pregnant and want to know whether my hypertension should be treated during pregnancy. Also, which medications are considered safe during pregnancy?*

A Your doctor should probably prescribe appropriate medication if and when your diastolic pressure exceeds 95. Once you are pregnant, you should be followed for possible preeclampsia. Methyldopa (e.g., Aldomet) and hydralazine (e.g., Apresoline) are still the drugs of choice during pregnancy.

In-Depth

Under normal circumstance, our heart beats about 60 to 80 times a minute. Blood pressure rises with each heartbeat and falls between beats when the heart relaxes. Your blood pressure can change from minute to minute depending on whether you are sitting or standing, at rest or engaged in some activity.

Normal blood pressure falls within a range. Healthy adult blood pressure is less than 120/80 mmHg. Blood pressure that stays between 140/90 mmHg or higher is considered high (hypertension). The first (higher) number represents the systolic pressure while the heart is beating. The second (lower) number represents the diastolic pressure when the heart is resting between beats.

About 5% to 10% of all pregnancies are complicated by hypertension. Chronic hypertension is elevated blood pressure (greater than 140/90 mmHg) before week 20 of pregnancy that persists beyond 6 weeks after the birth of the baby. Essential hypertension (hypertension that develops without apparent cause) accounts for 90% of these cases, while secondary causes, such as kidney diseases and endocrine and connective tissue disorders, are responsible for the rest.

Preeclampsia

Preeclampsia is a complex clinical syndrome characterized by hypertension, edema (swelling), and proteinuria (protein in the urine) that appears after the 20th week of the pregnancy in women who previously had normal blood pressure.

Women with chronic hypertension are at increased risk mainly for preeclampsia and abruptio placentae (premature detachment of the placenta). Preeclampsia, especially in its severe form, can lead to maternal convulsions, central nervous system hemorrhage, defects in the body's blood clotting mechanism, pulmonary edema, congestive heart failure, liver function abnormalities, and kidney failure.

The chief requirements for successful management of preeclampsia are early diagnosis, close follow-up, and timely delivery. Because severe preeclampsia might result in rapid deterioration of both mother and fetus, prompt delivery is indicated in cases of imminent eclampsia, multiorgan dysfunction, and fetal distress that occur after the 34th week of pregnancy.

The medical literature is far from consistent on whether antihypertensive therapy is indicated for mild, uncomplicated cases of preeclampsia. While some studies have shown antihypertensive therapy to have benefits for proteinuria, progression to severe disease, and neonatal respiratory syndrome, others failed to demonstrate any effect. In cases of severe or complicated preeclampsia, on the other hand, antihypertensive therapy is mandatory to ensure better outcomes.

Available Medications

Several studies have confirmed that hydralazine use during pregnancy (either alone or with other antihypertensive drugs) is not associated with congenital malformations. Although some anecdotal case reports have linked hydralazine with some adverse effects, the number of such cases is very small.

 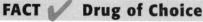

There is also a growing body of research that may support the careful use of other medications to treat hypertension during pregnancy. For example, in a prospective controlled study, Motherisk reported on the pregnancy outcome of 78 women who had been exposed to calcium channel blockers in the first trimester. Those who took calcium channel blockers did not have higher rates of major malformations or perinatal complications than those who did not. Although these data are reassuring, larger cohorts will have to be analyzed before safety can be established. Maternal hypertension was the most important factor responsible for low birth-weight babies in the group taking calcium channel blockers.

Other studies have looked at the use of nifedipine (e.g., Adalat) during the second and third trimesters of pregnancy and found that it lowers maternal blood pressure without affecting fetal heart rate or blood pressure. Nifedipine's efficacy and low toxicity are expected to make it a much-used agent during pregnancy.

SAFETY/RISK ❖ Beta-Blockers

Beta-blockers are also being studied and so far it appears that they have no major teratogenic effects on humans. However, there are still concerns about their possible association with other adverse effects. For that reason, though most newborns have not shown any adverse clinical signs, fetuses exposed in utero to beta-blockers should be closely followed with ultrasounds, and newborns should be followed for potential bradycardia (slow heart beat) or hypoglycemia (low glucose in the blood).

Diuretic therapy may be indicated particularly for chronically hypertensive pregnant women with salt-sensitive hypertension or with evidence of left ventricular diastolic dysfunction. Results of nine randomized trials of diuretic use during pregnancy demonstrated that these agents protected women with hypertension and left ventricular dysfunction against development of preeclampsia. Diuretic therapy should be discontinued, however, if there is evidence of either preeclampsia or retarded fetal growth.

Contraindicated Medications

Exposure to ACE inhibitors during the second and third trimesters of pregnancy is associated with development of kidney failure in the fetus and other fetal complications. However, several surveillance studies have shown no association with increased risk of structural malformations or major teratogenic effect where the use of ACE inhibitors was stopped during the first trimester. That should be encouraging news for women who were taking ACE inhibitors at the time of conception but stopped during the first trimester when they learned that they were pregnant. (Remember: about 50% of all pregnancies are unplanned.) Newborns exposed to ACE inhibitors *in utero* should nonetheless be closely monitored for kidney function and blood pressure.

Managing Hypothyroidism

Q I'm pregnant and taking levothyroxine for hypothyroidism. My doctor has prescribed iron because I was anemic, but I continue to be weak and to have high levels of thyroid-stimulating hormone (TSH). Increasing my dose of levothyroxine did not seem to affect my TSH levels.

A Many women need higher doses of levothyroxine during pregnancy. Your doctor should continue to monitor your TSH levels carefully and be aware that iron given during pregnancy might form an insoluble complex with thyroxine in the gestational tract.

In-Depth

Maternal hypothyroidism affects between 0.19% and 2.5% of pregnancies, depending on race and geographic area. Many hypothyroid women (>70%) have anovulatory cycles (menstrual bleeding occurs but no egg is produced) and, when they conceive, have high rates of fetal loss in the first trimester (more than twice as many spontaneous abortions as normal women). Studies have shown that the fetuses of hypothyroid women have 10% to 20% more congenital anomalies, 20% more perinatal mortality (stillbirth and neonatal death), and 50% to 60% higher rates of impaired mental and physical development than those of non-affected women. Maternal complications include overt anemia, preeclampsia, abruptio placentae, cardiac dysfunction, and hypertension.

Effects of Hypothyroidism

Two studies have shown that low maternal thyroid hormone concentrations during early gestation might be associated with substantially lower IQ scores in children when tested at school age. Also, the children of hypothyroid women with high concentrations of TSH due to inadequate doses of levothyroxine have impaired psychological development compared with carefully matched control children. It is important to note that the IQs of children of women who had high TSH concentrations but did not exhibit clinical hypothyroidism were also affected. Eventually, many of these women developed clinical disease.

FACT ✔ **Drug of Choice**

All hypothyroid women require daily, lifelong treatment. Levothyroxine is the treatment of choice. Administration of levothyroxine alone is preferable because the hormone content of the synthetic drug is more reliably standardized; this medication has replaced desiccated thyroid tablets as the mainstay of therapy.

When to Take Levothyroxine

The best time to take levothyroxine is early in the morning on an empty stomach. Some women, particularly during the first trimester, might not be able to tolerate medications at that time of day due to morning sickness, and it is probably better to allow them to take levothyroxine later when they are not experiencing nausea and vomiting. Insisting on administration of the medication early in the morning (regardless of patients' symptoms) might lead to skipping this important medication too often.

Many pregnant women take ferrous sulfate during pregnancy. This medication could form insoluble ferric-thyroxin complexes in the gastrointestinal tract and result in reduced absorption of levothyroxine. That is why these two drugs should be taken at least 2 hours apart.

SAFETY/RISK ❖ **Maintain Thyroid Levels**

Maintenance of thyroid hormone levels within the normal range is vital for pregnant woman to ensure optimal maternal and fetal health. Improved outcomes of pregnancy in hypothyroid women have been achieved through efforts to identify and treat these women. Normal thyroid gland function must be reached and maintained in a timely fashion. Levothyroxine is the treatment of choice. Levels of both TSH and thyroid hormone need to be monitored periodically, and concurrent administration of other medications should be carefully followed.

Guide to Safety/Risk of Prescription Drugs in Pregnancy

The information we provide here is not meant to replace the advice of your doctor. It is simply meant to make you better informed. Better-informed individuals tend to make better decisions concerning their health.

NOTES ON USING THIS CHART

1. The following table lists many medications and what we know about their use in pregnancy. The evidence that exists on the medication 'grades' the information given here. This evidence may change as more research becomes available.

2. With thousands of medications on the market, it is impossible to include them all here. If you use a medication that is not on this list, you may want to contact a teratogen information service near you. Their contact numbers are listed at the back of the book in the "Resources" section.

3. Often a medication is a mixture of two or more active ingredients, so it will be important to check out all ingredients. Read you prescription label carefully and consult with your physician or pharmacist if in doubt.

4. The generic (scientific-chemical) name of the medication appears in bold. The medication's different commercial names are shown in roman or regular type.

5. Read your prescription carefully, noting the generic name of the medication. If the generic name is not listed, ask your pharmacist or physician.

DRUG NAME	COMMON USE	FETAL SAFETY	REMARKS
Abacavir Ziagen, Combination form: Trizivir	• HIV1 Infections causing AIDs	Probably Safe	It is important to treat HIV to ensure maternal health and prevent fetal infection.
Acarbose Prandase, Precose, Glucobay	• Type 2 (adult) Diabetes Mellitus	Possibly Safe	Mother's diabetes needs to be controlled. Drug of choice in pregnancy is insulin.
Acetaminophen Abenol, Tempra, Tylenol, Atasol preparation, Pediatrix, Combination Form: Triaminic Cold, Nighttime Relief, Dimetapp, Dristan, Sinutab, Parafon Forte, Robaxacet, Methoxacet, Endocet, APAP, Actifed, Anexsia, Benadryl Cold, Lortab, Lorcet, etc.	• Pain • Fever	Safe	Drug of choice for pain and fever in pregnancy.
Acetazolamide Diamox	• Hypertension • Edema (swelling due to water retention)	Probably Safe	
Acetohexamide Dymelor	• Type 2 (adult) Diabetes Milletus	Unclear	Mother's diabetes needs to be controlled. Drug of choice in pregnancy is insulin.
Acitretin Soriatane	• Acne	**UNSAFE**	Causes malformations of the brain, ear, and internal organs.
Acyclovir Zovirax	• Viruses: Herpes Simplex, Varicella (Chicken Pox)	Probably Safe	Herpes simplex can cause serious neonatal morbidity, so the drug should be used if mother has vaginal herpes.
Adenosine Adenocard	• Antiarrhythmic (Irregular Heart Beats)	Unclear	

DRUG NAME	COMMON USE	FETAL SAFETY	REMARKS
Albendazole Valbazen, Zentel	• Certain Worms	Possibly Safe	The drug is poorly absorbed from the gut. Absorption increases with fatty meals.
Albuterol Salbutamol, Proventil, Ventolin, Airet, Volmax	• Premature Labor Prevention	Probably Safe	
Alfentanil (narcotic) Alfenta, Opioids	• Severe Pain •	Probably Safe	
Allopurinol Zyloprim	• Gout (and other conditions with high uric acid)	Possibly Safe	
Alprazolam (a Benzodiazepine from the Valium family) Xanax, Xanax TS, Benzodiazepines	• Anxiety • Sleeplessness	Possibly Safe	Baby may experience withdrawal when used near term. There is a marginal risk for clefts. Mother should have LII ultrasound.
Alteplase Cathflo, Activase	• Blood Clotting	Unclear	
Amantadine Edantadine, Symmetrel Anti-Parkinson	• Anti-Parkinson • Influenza Virus	Unclear	
Amikacin Amikin	• Antibiotic	Probably Safe	
Amiloride Midamor, Moduretic; Combination Form: Novamilor, APO-Amilizide	• Hypertension • Fluid Retention (diuretic)	Probably Safe	
Aminogluthetamide Cytadren	• Antiepileptic	Unclear	
Aminopterin	• Anticancer	**UNSAFE**	Causes fetal defects, especially in first trimester.

DRUG NAME	COMMON USE	FETAL SAFETY	REMARKS
Para-Aminosalicylic Acid Nemasol, PAS	• Tuberculosis	Possibly Safe	Tuberculosis must be treated in pregnant women without delay.
Amitriptyline Triavil, HCL: Elavil, Etrafon-A, EndepLimbitrol	• Depression	Safe	Baby may experience withdrawal if used near term.
Amlodipine Norvasc	• Hypertension	Probably Safe	
Ammonium Chloride Combination Form: Balminil, Cheracol, Hycomine	• Alkalosis (high pH in the blood)	Probably Safe	
Amoxapine Asendin	• Antidepressant	Probably Safe	
Amoxicillin Amoxil, Augmentin, Moxilin, Wymox	• Antibiotic	Safe	
Amphetamine Adderall, Biphetamine	• Appetite Suppression	Possibly Safe	
Amphotericin B Fungizone, Abelcet, Ambisome	• Infectious Fungal	Possibly Safe	
Ampicillin Omnipen, Unasyn	• Antibiotic	Safe	
Amprenavir Agenerase	• HIV1 Infections causing AIDs	Possibly Safe	
Amyl Nitrate	• Angina Pectoris	Unclear	
Aprotinin Trasylol	• Blood Clotting Treatment • Blood Loss Prevention	Possibly Safe	
Asparaginase Elspar	• Anticancer	**UNSAFE IN FIRST TRIMESTER**	

DRUG NAME	COMMON USE	FETAL SAFETY	REMARKS
Aspartame Nutrasweet	• Sweetener	Safe when used in moderation	
Aspirin ASA, ASACOL, Alka-Seltzer, Axotal, Damason-P, Darvon, Ecotrin, Excedrin, Fiorinal, Norgesic, Halfprin, Percodan, Talwin, ACUPRIN	• Pain • Fever • Inflammation	Probably Safe	May cause closure of the fetal vessel (ductus arteriosus) with high dose near terms.
Astemizole Hismanal	• Non-sedating Antihistamine	Probably Safe	
Atorvastatin Lipitor	• Lower Cholesterol Levels	Unclear	
Atracurium Tracrium	• Surgery (to relax muscles)	Possibly Safe	
Atropine	• Heart Rate (to increase) • Anticholinergic Signs (to counteract)	Possibly Safe	
Azathioprine Imuran, Apo-Azathioprine, Gen-Azathioprine, Ratio-Azathioprine	• Organ Transplant • Arthritis • Lupus • Inflammatory Bowel Disease	Possibly Safe	
Azithromycin Zithromax (Z-pak)	• Antibiotic	Probably Safe	
Beclomethasone (Beclomethasone Dipropionate) Beclovent, Beconase, Vancenase	• AQ Nasal Spray C • Bronchial Asthma (prevention and treatment) • Allergic Rhinitis	Possibly Safe	Unlike systemic corticosteroids (given by tablets or ingestions). No fetal adverse effect described with inhaled corticosteroids.

DRUG NAME	COMMON USE	FETAL SAFETY	REMARKS
Beta-carotene (precursor of vitamin A) Antiox	• Vitamin A Deficiency	Probably Safe	
Betamethasone	• Inflammation • Collagen-like Autoimmune Diseases • Fetal Lung Maturity	Possibly Safe In first trimester may increase risk of oral cleft (cleft palate and lip)	Beneficial to mature fetal lungs, decreases respiratory distress syndrome and intracranial hemorrhages.
Bleomycin Sulfate Blenoxane, Faulding	• Anticancer	**UNSAFE**	Causes fetal malformations in first trimester.
Bromocriptine Mesylate Parlodel	• Infertility • Hyperprolactinemia	Possibly Safe	
Brompheniramine Maleate Bromfed Capsules, Dimetane-DC Cough Syrup, ULTRABROM Capsules, Dimetapp-C syrup, Lodrane LD Capsules, Poly-Histine CS, Touro A&H Capsules	• Antihistamine	Possibly Safe	
Budesonide Rhinocort Nasal Inhaler, Cortiscotics: Eye Ear Nose, Pulmicort Nebuamp	• Asthma Prophylaxis • Allergic Rhinitis	Probably Safe	
Bupropion Hydrochloride Wellbutrin Tablets, Zyban	• Antidepressant • Smoking Cessation	Possibly Safe	
Buspirone Hydrochloride Buspar	• Anxiety	Possibly Safe	

DRUG NAME	COMMON USE	FETAL SAFETY	REMARKS
Busulfan Myleran, Busulfex	• Anticancer	**UNSAFE**	Can cause congenital malformations.
Butalbital Barbiturates, Axotal, Floricet Tablets, Fiorinal Cap/Tab, Phrenilin Forte Capsules, Sedapap Tablets, Bupap Tablets, Esgic Cap/Tab	• Sleeplessness • Anxiety	Possibly Safe	
Caffeine Cafergot Tablets, Ergodryl, Norgesic, Caffeine/ASA (Midol Regular), Caffeine/ASA/Butalbital (Trianal, Fiorinal)	• Stimulant	Probably Safe	Use less than 150 mg(d) per day (no more than 1 to 2 cups of average coffee).
Calciterol (Vitamin D) Capoten, Capozide, ACE Inhibitor, Apo-capto, Novo-Captopril	• Vitamin D Deficiency	Probably Safe	
Captopril Capoten, Capozide, ACE inhibitor, Apo-capto, Novo-Captopril	• Antihypertensive	**UNSAFE**	Can cause renal failure in baby and inhibits the development of the skull. Women on captopril should be switched to other antihypertensive drugs.
Carbamazepine Tegretol, Apo-Carbomazepine, Novo-Carbamaze, Taro-Carbamazepine	• Antiepileptic	**UNSAFE**	Causes spina bifida and other neural tube defects in around 1% of exposed fetuses in early pregnancy. Rule out neural tube defects by detailed ultrasound and maternal alfa-fetoproteins.
Carbenicillin Indanyl Sodium Geocillin	• Antibiotic	Unclear	Minimal experience in human pregnancy.

DRUG NAME	COMMON USE	FETAL SAFETY	REMARKS
Carvedilol Coreg	• Hypertension	Probably Safe	
Cefaclor Ceclor Pulvules & Suspension, Apo-Cefaclor, Novo-Cefaclor	• Antibiotic	Safe	
Cefadroxil Duricef	• Antibiotic	Safe	
Cefamandole Nafate Mandol	• Antibiotic	Safe	
Cefatrizine	• Antibiotic	Safe	
Cefazolin Sodium Kefzol, Ancef Injection	• Antibiotic	Safe	
Cefepime Maxipime	• Antibiotic	Safe	
Cefixime Suprax	• Antibiotic	Safe	
Cefmetazole Sodium Zefazone	• Antibiotic	Safe	
Cefonicid Sodium Monocid	• Antibiotic	Safe	
Cefoperazone Cefobid	• Antibiotic	Safe	
Cefotaxime Sodium Claforan	• Antibiotic	Safe	
Cefoxitin Mefoxin	• Antibiotic	Safe	
Cefprozil Cefzil	• Antibiotic	Safe	
Ceftazidime Fortaz, Tazidime, Ceptaz Tazicef	• Antibiotic	Safe	

DRUG NAME	COMMON USE	FETAL SAFETY	REMARKS
Ceftriaxone Rocephin	• Antibiotic	Safe	
Cefuroxime Axetil: Ceftin, Cefuroxime; Sodium: Kefurox Zinacef	• Antibiotic	Safe	
Celecoxib Celebrex	• Pain • Inflammation	Unclear	
Cephalexin Keflex, Apo-Cephalex, Novo-Lexin	• Antibiotic	Safe	
Cephalothin Keflin	• Antibiotic	Safe	
Cephradine	• Antibiotic	Safe	
Cerivastatin Baycol	• Cholesterol Lowering	Unknown	
Cetirizine Zyrtec, Reactine, Apo-Cetirizine	• Non-sedating Antihistamine	Probably Safe	
Chenodiol Chenix, Chenodeoxycholic Acid	• Dissolve Gallstone	**UNSAFE**	May cause liver damage to fetus.
Chloral Hydrate Aquachloral Supprettes	• Sleeplessness • Anxiety	Possibly Safe	
Chlorambucil Leukeran	• Anticancer	**UNSAFE**	
Chlordiazepoxide (Hydrochloride) Librax, Librium	• Sleeplessness • Anxiety	Possibly Safe	
Chlorhexidine (Gluconate) Betasept Surgical Scrub, Peridex (Acetate): Bactigras	• Antiseptic	Safe	For local use only.

DRUG NAME	COMMON USE	FETAL SAFETY	REMARKS
Chlorothiazide Aldoclor, Diupres, Diuril	• Hypertension • Fluid Retention	Possibly Safe	
Chlorpheniramine Malate: Chlor-Tripolon, Triaminic Cold, Dimetapp Nighttime Cold; Polistirex: Tussionex Pennkinetic; Tannate: Atrohist Pediatric, Ricobid Rynatuss, Triotann	• Antihistamine	Safe	
Chlorpromazine (Hydrochloride) Largactil, Thorazine	• Schizophrenia • Sedation • Vomiting	Probably Safe	
Chlorpropamide Diabinese, Sulfonylureas, Apo-Chlorpropamide	• Type 2 (adult) Diabetes Mellitus	Possibly Safe	No malformation, but neonatal hypoglycemia may occur. Drug of choice is insulin.
Cholestyramine Questran, Novo-Cholamine	• Excess Bile Acids • Itching Prevention	Possibly Safe	
Cidofovir	• HIV1 Infections causing AIDS • Cytomegalo Infections	Possibly Safe	It is important to treat HIV to ensure maternal health and prevent neonatal infection.
Cimetidine Tagamet, Apo-Cimetidine, Novo-Cimetine, Nu-Cimet	• Peptic Ulcers	Probably Safe	
Cinoxacin Cinobac	• Antibiotic	Unknown	
Ciprofloxacin Cipro, Cipro HC: Ciloxan	• Antibiotic	Probably Safe	
Cisapride Propulsid	• Gastrointestinal Reflux	Probably Safe	

DRUG NAME	COMMON USE	FETAL SAFETY	REMARKS
Cisplatin Platinol	• Anticancer	**UNSAFE**	
Citalopram Celexa	• Antidepressant	Possibly Safe	
Clarithromycin Biaxin, Biaxin XL, Biaxin Bid	• Antibiotic	Possibly Safe	
Clavulanic Acid Clavulin, APO-Amoxi-Clav	• Antibiotic	Probably Safe	
Clemastine Tavist	• Antihistamine	Safe	
Clindamycin Cleocin, Dalacin C, Sabex	• Antibiotic	Probably Safe	
Clomiphene Clomid, Serophene	• Fertility Agent	Unknown	No apparent evidence of malformations, but not sufficient safety data.
Clomipramine Anafranil, Apo-Clomipramine, Novo-Clopamin	• Antidepressant	Probably Safe	Possible withdrawal.
Clonazepam (a Benzodiazepine from the Valium family) Klonopin, Novo-Clonazepam, Rivotril	• Anxiety • Sleeplessness • Seizures	Probably Safe	Baby may experience withdrawal if used near term.
Clonidine Catapres, Dixarit, Combipres, Apo-Clonidine, Novo-Clonidine	• Hypertension • Pain	Possibly Safe	

DRUG NAME	COMMON USE	FETAL SAFETY	REMARKS
Clotrimazole Canesten Topical, Canesten Vaginal, Clotrimaderm, Lotrimin, Lotrisone, Mycelex OTC Cream, Clotrimazole/betameth asone: Lotriderm	• Fungal Infections	Possibly Safe	
Cloxacillin Apo-Cloxi, Novo-Cloxi, Nu-Cloxi	• Antibiotic	Safe	
Clozapine Clozaril, Rhoxa-clozapinel	• Schizophrenia	Possibly Safe	
Codeine Phosphate: Opioids, Ratio-Codeine; Phosphate/Acetamino-phen: Ratio-Entec, Tylenol No. 4 with Codeine	• Pain	Probably Safe	Baby may suffer withdrawal when used near term.
Colchicine	• Gout	**UNSAFE**	Insufficient data on safety.
Coumarin Coumadin, Warfarin, Anisindione, Dicumarol, Acenocoumarol, Phenindione, Diphenindione, Phenprocoumon	• Blood Clotting Prevention	**UNSAFE**	Causes congenital malformations when taken in the first trimester: dwarfism, bone, brain damage. Should not be used during the first trimester and near birth.
Cromolyn Sodium Gastrocrom, Nasalcrom Nasal Solution, Sodium Cromoglycate	• Asthma Prevention	Probably Safe	
Cyclizine	• Antihistamine	Safe	
Cyclobenzaprine HCL: Flexeril, Apo-cyclobenzaprine, Novo-cycloprine	• Muscle Relaxation	Probably Safe	

DRUG NAME	COMMON USE	FETAL SAFETY	REMARKS
Cyclophosphamide Cytoxan, Procytox, NEOSAR Lyophilize	• Anticancer	**UNSAFE**	Can cause congenital malformation; most risk in first trimester.
Cyclosporine Neoral, Rhoxal-cyclosporine, Sandimmune	• Organ Transplant	Probably Safe	
Cyproheptadine Periactin	• Antihistamine • Antiserotonin	Probably Safe	
Cytarabine Cytosar-U, Cytosine Arabinoside, Cytarabine Liposome (Depocyt)	• Anticancer	**UNSAFE**	Can cause congenital malformations; most risk in first trimester.
Dacarbazine DTIC, DTIC-Dome	• Anticancer	**UNSAFE**	Can cause congenital malformation; most risk in first trimester.
Dactinomycin Cosmegen, Actinomycin D	• Anticancer	**UNSAFE**	Can cause congenital malformations; most risk in first trimester.
Dalteparin Sodium Fragmin, Heparins: low molecular weight	• Blood Clotting Prevention	Safe	
Danaparoid Sodium Organ-DVT, Organ-HIT	• Blood Clotting Prevention	Safe	
Danazol (male sex hormone) Cyclomen, Danocrine	• Endometriosis • Fibrocystic Breast Disease	**UNSAFE**	May cause masculine changes in fetus. Should not be used in pregnancy.
Dantrolene Sodium Danyrium	• Muscle Relaxant for Malignant Hyperthermia	Possibly Safe	
Dapsone Dapson USP	• Lepra Malaria	Possibly Safe	
Daunorubicin (HCL) Cerubidine, Daunomycin	• Anticancer	**UNSAFE**	Can cause congenital malformations; most risk in first trimester.

DRUG NAME	COMMON USE	FETAL SAFETY	REMARKS
Deferoxamine Desferal, PMS-Deferoxamine	• Iron Chelation	Possibly Safe	
Delavirdine Mesylate Rescriptor	• HIV1 Infections causing AIDs	Possibly Safe	It is important to treat HIV to ensure maternal health and prevent neonatal infection.
Desipramine (HCL) Norpramin, Novo-Desipramine, Apo-Desipramine	• Antidepressant	Safe	
Dexamethasone Cortcosteroids: Eye Ear Nose, Decadron, Dexasone, Maxidex; Combination Form: Tobradex, Dalalone D.P. , Decadron-LA,Dexacort, NeoDecadron, Hexadrol	• Asthma • Inflammatory Bowel Syndrome • Autoimmune Conditions • Pregnancy Related Issues	**MAY BE UNSAFE IN FIRST TRIMESTER**	May increase risk for oral cleft in first trimester; cleft lip and palate; reduced fetal head circumference. Reduces respiratory distress syndrome by maturing the fetal lung. Decreases fetal morbidity from intracranial hemorrhages; increases survival of preterm infants.
Dexfenfluramine Fenfluramine	• Appetite Suppressor	Possibly Safe	
Dextromethorphan Benylin DM, Balminil DM; Children, Koffex DM, Combination Form: Tylenol Cough, Balminil Night-Time, Dimetapp DM Cough & Cold, Triaminic Cold & Cough, Dimetane-DX, Humibid DM, Fenesin DM, Sudafed Cold & Cough	• Cough	Probably Safe	

DRUG NAME	COMMON USE	FETAL SAFETY	REMARKS
Diazepam Valium, APO-Diazepam, Benzodiazepines, Diazemuls, Diastat	• Sleeplessness • Anxiety	Possibly Safe	Baby may experience withdrawal when used near term. Marginal risk of oral cleft.
Diazoxide Hyperstat, Proglycem	• Hypertension	Unclear	May decrease maternal blood pressure severely. Should be used cautiously in several hypertensions.
Diclectin Doxylamine Succinate/Pyridoxine Hydrochloride	• Antiemetic for Morning Sickness	Safe	
Diclofenac Voltaren, Cataflam	• Inflammation • Pain	Probably Safe	
Dicloxacillin Pathocil, Dynapen	• Antibiotic	Safe	
Dicyclomine Bentylol, Lomine, Bentyl	• Vomiting and Nausea	Safe	
Didanosine DDI, Videx, Videx EC	• HIV1 Infections causing AIDs	Possibly Safe	It is important to treat HIV to ensure maternal health and prevent neonatal infection.
Digitalis Crystodigin	• Heart Rate Irregularities • Heart Failure	Safe	May be used to treat heart conditions in the fetus.
Diltiazem (HCL) Cardizem, Tiazac, Dilacor	• Angina Pectoris	Possibly Safe	
Dimenhydrinate Gravol, DMH-Syrup	• Antihistamine	Safe	

DRUG NAME	COMMON USE	FETAL SAFETY	REMARKS
Diphenhydramine Benadryl, Allerdryl, Allernix, Nytol, Simply Sleep, Unisom Extra Strength, Actifed Allergy (Daytime/Nighttime), Actifed Sinus, Tylenol Allergy Sinus, Tylenol Flu Nighttime, Dytuss	• Antihistamine	Safe	
Diphenoxylate Lomotil	• Antidiarrheal	Possibly Safe	
Dipyridamole Persantine, Novo-Dipiradol	• Dilating Blood Vessels	Unknown	
Disopyramide Rythmodan	• Heartbeat Irregularities	Possibly Safe	
Disulfiram Antabuse	• Alcohol Drinking Prevention	Unclear	
Docusate Sodium Dialose, Diocto, Hemaspan, Prenate, Colace, Selax, Soflax	• Laxative	Probably Safe	
Doxepin (HCL) Adapin, Sinequan, Zonalon Cream, Apo-Doxepin, Novo-Doxepin	• Antidepressant	Safe	
Doxorubicin Adriamycin PFS, Adriamycin RDF, Rubex Liposome: Caelyx, Myocet	• Anticancer	**UNSAFE**	Can cause congenital malformations; risk mostly in first trimester.
Doxycycline Doryx, Vibramycin, Bio-Tab, Vibra-Tabs, Doxycin, Novo-Doxuylin, Apo-Doxy	• Antibiotic	**UNSAFE**	May stain fetal teeth and affect their growth; risk only after teeth buds begin to form (after 8 weeks).

DRUG NAME	COMMON USE	FETAL SAFETY	REMARKS
Doxylamine Unisome Nighttime Sleep Aid; Combination Form: Diclectin, Dalmacole, ratio-Calmydone, Tylenol Sinus Extra Strength, Mersyndol with Codeine	• Antihistamine for Morning Sickness	Safe	
Droperidol Innovar, Inapsine	• Schizophrenia • Vomiting	Probably Safe	
Efavirenz Sustiva	• HIV1 Infections causing AIDs	Possibly Safe	It is important to treat HIV to ensure maternal health and prevent neonatal infection.
Enalapril Vaseretic, Vasotec	• Hypertension	**UNSAFE**	Neonatal renal damage, lack of development of skull, neonatal death.
Encainide	• Heartbeat Problems	Possibly Safe	Used also to treat heart beat problems in fetus.
Enoxacin	• Antibiotic	Possibly Safe	
Enoxaparin Lovenox, Lovenox HP, Heparins	• Blood Clotting Prevention	Probably Safe	
Ephedrine (HCL) Quadrinal, Broncholate Softgels, Broncholate Syrup, Mudrane Tablets, Mudrane GG	• Asthma • Allergies • Upper Respiratory Tract Infection	Possibly Safe	
Epinephrine (HCL) Adrenalin, Vaponefrin, Epipen, Epipen Jr, Ana-Kit Anaphylaxis	• Shock • Glaucoma • Allergic Reaction • Asthma • Nasal Congestion	Possibly Safe	
Epirubicin Pharmorubicin PFS	• Anticancer	**UNSAFE**	Can cause congenital malformations; most risk in first trimester.

DRUG NAME	COMMON USE	FETAL SAFETY	REMARKS
Epoprostenol Sodium Flolan	• Dilating Blood Vessels • Primary Pulmonary Hypertension	Probably Safe	
Eprosartan Teveten	• Hypertension	**UNSAFE**	Unknown potential risk for renal damage to newborn; should be switched to another drug in pregnancy.
Erbumine Coversyl	• Hypertension	**UNSAFE**	Can cause renal shutdown and death in baby, and skull anomalies; should be switched to another antihypertensive drug.
Ergotamine Combination Form: Cafergot-PB, Bellergal Spacetabs, Ergodryl	• Migraine	**UNSAFE**	Should be avoided because it causes uterine contractions.
Erythromycin Erythrocin, Liosone, Eryzole, E.E.S Eryped Drops, Akne-mycin Ointment, Benzamycin Topical Gel, E-Mycin Tablets, Emgel, ERYC, Erycette, Ilotycin Ophthalmic, Pediazole, Theramycin Z Topical, Erygel, Erymax, Erythra-Derm, Liotycin Gluceptate	• Antibiotic	Safe	
Erythropoitin Eprex	• Red Blood Cell Production	Probably Safe	
Esmolol Brevibloc	• Hypertension • Heartbeat Irregularities	Unclear	

DRUG NAME	COMMON USE	FETAL SAFETY	REMARKS
Estradiol Climara, Estraderm, Estradot, Vivelle, Estrace, Estrogel, Oesclim, Vagifem, Estalis, Delestrogen, Estalis-Sequi, Estracomb	• Estrogenic Sex Hormone	Probably Safe	Large studies failed to show risk when used as recommended in the 'pill'.
Estrogens (conjugated) Premarin, PMB 200/400	• Estrogenic Sex Hormones	Probably Safe	Large studies failed to show risk when used as recommended in the 'pill'.
Ethambutol Etibi, Myambutol	• Tuberculosis	Probably Safe	Tuberculosis in pregnancy must be treated effectively.
Ethinyl Estradiol Combination Form: Diane, Marvelon, Ortho-Cept, Demulen, Alesse 21/ 28, Min-Ovral, Triphasil, Triquilar, Brevicon, Synphasi, FemHRT, Cyclin, Tri-Cyclen, Brevicon, Demulen, Desogen, Levlen, Loestrin, Lo/Oval, Modicon, Nordette, Ortho-Novum, Ortho Tri-Cyclen, Ovcon, Triphasil, Nelova	• Estrogenic Sex Hormone	Safe	Large studies failed to show risk when used as recommended in the 'pill'.
Ethosuximide Zarontin	• Antiepileptic	Possibly Safe	
Ethotoin Peganone	• Antiepileptic	Unclear	Theoretically may cause fetal hydantoin syndrome; brain, face, and other malformations.
Etodolac Utradol, Apo-Etodolac	• Inflammation Arthritis • Pain	Possibly Safe	

DRUG NAME	COMMON USE	FETAL SAFETY	REMARKS
Etoposide Vepesid	• Anticancer	**UNSAFE**	Can cause congenital malformations; risk mostly in first trimester.
Etretinate Tegison	• Psoriasis	**UNSAFE**	Can cause congenital malformations of the brain, ears, face, and other organs.
Famciclovir Famvir	• Herpes Simplex 1 & 2 • Chicken Pox	Possibly Safe	
Famotidine Pepcid	• Peptic Ulcer	Possibly Safe	
Felodipine Plendil Extended-Release	• Hypertension	Possibly Safe	
Fenfluramine Pondimin	• Appetite Control	Unclear	
Fenoprofen Nalfon	• Pain • Inflammation	Probably Safe	
Fentanyl Duragesic, Opioids	• Acute Pain • Anesthesia for Surgery	Possibly Safe	When used near term, the baby may experience withdrawal from this narcotic analgesic.
Flecainide Acetate Fleet	• Heart Rate Problems	Possibly Safe	Used to treat heart rate problems in the fetus.
Fluconazole Diflucan	• Fungal Infections	Possibly Safe	
Fluorouracil Efudex, Fluoroplex	• Anticancer	**UNSAFE**	Can cause congenital malformation; most risk in first trimester.
Fluoxetine (HCL) Prozac	• Antidepressant	Probably Safe	It is important to treat depression in pregnancy.

DRUG NAME	COMMON USE	FETAL SAFETY	REMARKS
Fluphenazine Prolixin	• Schizophrenia • Vomiting	Probably Safe	
Flurazepam (belongs to the Valium family) Dalmane	• Sleeplessness • Anxiety	Possibly Safe	
Flurbiprofen Ansaid	• Pain • Inflammation	Probably Safe	
Fluvastatin Sodium Lescol	• Cholesterol Production Prevention	Unknown	
Fluvoxamine Luvox	• Antidepressant	Probably Safe	
Furosemide Lasix	• Diuretic (for fluid retention)	Possibly Safe	
Gabapentin Neurontin, Novo-Gabapentin, Apo-Gabapentin	• Antiepileptic	Unknown	
Ganciclovir Cytovene	• Herpes Virus Infection • Cytomegalovirus	Unknown	
Gatifloxacin Tequin, Fluoroquinolones	• Antibiotic	Unknown	
Gentamicin Garamycin, Alcomicin, G-myticin Cream; Combination Form: Garasone Ophthalmic Drop, SAB-Pentasone, Valisone-G	• Antibiotic	Possibly Safe	
Glipizide Glucotrol	• Type 2 (adult) Diabetes Mellitus	Unknown	Possibly no increased malformation rates; may cause neonatal hypoglycemia. Insulin is the drug of choice for diabetes mellitus in pregnancy.

DRUG NAME	COMMON USE	FETAL SAFETY	REMARKS
Glyburide Diabeta, Glynase Pres Tab, Micronase, Glibenclamide, Euglucon, Gen-Gybe, Ratio-Glyburide, Sulfonylureas	• Type 2 (adult) Diabetes Mellitus	Unknown	Possibly no increased malformation rates. The drug does not appear to cross from the mother to the fetus.
Gold Myochrysine	• Rheumatoid (Joint Inflammation) Diseases	Possibly Safe	
Granisetron Kytril	• Vomiting	Unknown	
Griseofulvin Fulvicin P/G, Fulvicin U/F Grifulvin V, Gris-PEG, Grisactin, Grisactin Ultra	• Fungal Infections	Unknown	
Guanethidine Esimil, Ismelin	• Hypertension	Unknown	Safety in first trimester unknown.
Haloperidol Haldol	• Schizophrenia • Strong Tranquilizer • Vomiting	Probably Safe	
Heparins Heparin Sodium: Hepalean, Hepalean-Lok, Heparin Leo, Hep-Lock	• Blood Clotting Prevention	Probably Safe	
Hexachlorophene PhisoHex	• Topical (skin) Antiseptic	Safe when used appropriately	
Hydralazine Apresoline, Novo-Hylazin, Nu-Hydral, Apo-Hydralazine	• Hypertension	Possibly Safe	

DRUG NAME	COMMON USE	FETAL SAFETY	REMARKS
Hydrocodone Bitartrate Anexsia, Codiclear DH, Damason-P, Duratuss HD, Hydrocet, Lorcet, Lortab, Vicodin, Anaplex HD, Azdone, Bancap HC, Codimal DH, Co-Gesic; Combination Form: Hycodan, Opioids, Hycomine, Hycomine-S, Polistirex: Tussionex	• Pain	Possibly Safe	Baby may experience withdrawal if used near term.
Hydrocortisone Acetasol HC, Cotenema, Cortisporin Ointment, Hydeocortone, Hytone Cream/Lotion, Penecorte Cream, Vytone Cream, Cortisol, Claratin Itch Skin Relief, Cortrate, Cortef Tablets, Cortenema, Cortiscosteroids: Eye Ear Nose, Cortoderm, Emo-Cort, Hycort, Prevex, HC, Sarna HC, Cortef Cream, Cortifoam, Hyderm, Rectogel HC, Pentamycin/HC, Fucidin H, Pramox HC, Proctofoam-HC, Anuzinc HC Plus, Anugesic-HC, Proctodan-HC, Uremol HC, Anuzinc HC, Anodan-HC, Anusol HC, Ratio-Hemcort-HC, Rivasol HC, Cortimyxin, Cortisporin Ointment, Vioform Hydrocortisone, Proctosedyl, Solu-Cortef, HydroVal	• Inflammation • Asthma • Autoimmune Diseases (e.g., lupus)	Probably Safe	May cause oral cleft (cleft palate or lip) in first trimester when used in oral doses.

DRUG NAME	COMMON USE	FETAL SAFETY	REMARKS
Hydroxychloroquine Plaquenil Sulfate	• Malaria • Rheumatoid Arthritis	Possibly Safe	
Hydroxyprogesterone Delalutin	• Female Sex Hormone	Probably Safe when part of the 'pill'	
Hydroxyurea Hydrea, Gen-Hydroxyurea	• Cancer • Sickle Cell Disease	**UNSAFE**	May cause congenital malformations.
Hydroxyzine Atarax, Marax, Vistaril, Novo-Hydroxyzin, Apo-Hydroxyzin	• Antihistamine	Possibly Safe	
Ibuprofen Advil, Motrin, Dristan Sinus, Apo-Ilbuprofen; Combination Form: Novo-Profen, Advil Cold & Sinus, Sudafed S, IBU-Tablets, IBU-TAB OTC	• Inflammation • Pain	Probably Safe	Near term may cause premature closure of the fetal vessel (ductus arteriosus).
Idarubicin Idamycin	• Cancer	**UNSAFE**	Can cause congenital malformations; most risk in first trimester.
Imipramine Tofranil-PM, Apo-Impipramine	• Depression	Probably Safe	Baby may experience withdrawal when used near term.
Indinavir Crixivan, Inocid	• HIV1 infection causing AIDs	Possibly Safe	It is important to treat HIV to ensure maternal health and prevent neonatal infection.
Indomethacin Indocin	• Pain • Inflammation	Possibly Safe	Near term may cause premature closure of the fetal vessel (ductus arteriosus).

DRUG NAME	COMMON USE	FETAL SAFETY	REMARKS
Insulin Human NPH: Humulin N, Novolin N, Human Regular: Humulin N, Humulin R, Novolin R, Velosulin Human, Novo-Rapid, Innovo, Humulin-L, Novolin Ge Lente, Iletin 11 Pork Lente, Humalog, Humulin, Humulin-U, Lente Iletin 11, Lente Insulin, Lente Purified Pork, Ultralente Insulin	• Diabetes Mellitus	Safe	
Interferon Alfa-2a: Roferon-A, Alfa-2b: Intron A, Alfa-2b/Ribavirin: Rebetron, Beta-1a: Avonex, Rebif, Actimmune, Beta-1b: Betaseron	• Hepatitis C • Cancer	Possibly Safe	Does not seem to cross from mother to baby.
Ipratropium Atrovent Inhalation, Novo-Ipramide, Nu-Ipratropium	• Asthma	Possibly Safe	
Irbesartan Avapro, Avalide	• Hypertension	**UNSAFE**	Theoretically may cause neonatal renal shutdown; should be switched to other medications in pregnancy.
Isoniazid INH, Isonicotine Acid Hydrazide, Isonicotinylhydrazide, Isotamine, PMS-Isoniazid; Combination Form: Isoniazid/Pyrazinamid/ Rifampin: Rifater	• Tuberculosis	Possibly Safe	

DRUG NAME	COMMON USE	FETAL SAFETY	REMARKS
Isopropamide Darbid	• Anticholinergic	Possibly Safe	
Isoproterenol (HCL) Isoprenaline, Isopropylaterenol Isopropylnoradre-naline	• Asthma • Upper Respiratory Infections	Possibly Safe	
Isotretinoin Accutane, Cis-retinoic, Accutane Roche, Isotrex	• Acne	**UNSAFE**	Can cause congenital malformation, including brain, ears, and internal organs. Should not be used by planning or pregnant women, or those having unprotected sex.
Itraconazole Sporanox	• Fungal Infections	Possibly Safe	
Ketamine Ketaler	• Anesthesia	Probably Safe	
Ketoconazole Ketoderm, Nizoral, Apo-Ketoconazole, Novo-Ketoconazole	• Fungal Infections	Probably Safe	
Ketoprofen Orudis-SR, Rhodis, Rhovail, Apo-Keto, Novo-Keto	• Pain • Inflammation	Probably Safe	At term may cause premature closure of the fetal vessel (ductus arteriosus).
Ketorolac Tromethamine Acular, Toradol, Apo-Ketorolac, Novo-Ketorolac	• Pain • Inflammation	Possibly Safe	At term may cause premature closure of the fetal vessel (ductus arteriosus).
Labetalol Trandate, Normodyne	• Hypertension	Probably Safe	
Levothyroxine	• Hypothyroidism	Safe	

DRUG NAME	COMMON USE	FETAL SAFETY	REMARKS
Lithium Carbonate Carbolith, Duralith, Lithane, Eskalith, Lithonate, Lithotabs	• Manic Depression	Probably Safe	In rare instances, can cause Epstein anomaly (heart malformation); can be used safely after first trimester.
Lomefloxacin Maxaquin	• Antibiotic	Possibly Safe	
Loperamide Imodium, Apo-Loperamide, Novo-Loperamide	• Diarrhea	Probably Safe	
Loratadine Claritin, Apo-Loratadine	• Antihistamine	Probably Safe	
Lorazepam (belongs to the Valium group) Ativan, Benzodiazepines, Novo-Lorazem	• Sleeplessness • Anxiety	Possibly Safe	Baby may experience withdrawal when used near term. There is a marginal risk for clefts. Mother should have LII ultrasound.
Losartan Cozaar, Hyzaar	• Hypertension	**UNSAFE**	May theoretically cause neonatal renal shutdown and neonatal death; should be switched to another antihypertensive drug.
Lovastatin Mevacor	• Cholesterol Lowering	Unknown	
Magnesium Sulfate Eldertonic, Eldercaps (Combination Form: Magnesium Sulfate/Benzocaine: Osmopak Plus)	• Seizures • Eclampsia	Safe	
Mebendazole Vermox	• Worm Infections	Unknown	
Meclizine (HCL) Antivert, Bonine, Histamethizine, Bonamine	• Antihistamine	Probably Safe	

DRUG NAME	COMMON USE	FETAL SAFETY	REMARKS
Meclofenamate Meclofenamic acid	• Pain • Inflammation	Probably Safe	Near term may cause premature closure of the fetal vessel (ductus arteriosus).
Medroxy-Progesterone Depo-Provera, Provera, Amen, Cycrin	• Female Sex Hormone	Probably Safe when used in the 'pill'	
Mefloquine Lariam	• Malaria	Possibly Safe	Important to treat maternal malaria in pregnancy.
Meperidine (HCL) Demerol, Mepegan, Pethidine HCL	• Acute Pain	Probably Safe	When used near term, the baby may exhibit withdrawal.
Meprobamate Miltown, PMB 200 and PMB, Equagesic, Equanil, Meprospan	• Sleeplessness • Anxiety	Possibly Safe	When used near term, the baby may exhibit withdrawal.
Mercaptopurine Purinethol (Tablets)	• Cancer • Inflammatory Bowel Disease • Organ Transplant	**UNSAFE**	May cause congenital malformation; most risk in first trimester.
Mesalamine Asacol Delayed-Release, Pentasa, Rowasa Rectal	• Inflammatory Bowel Disease	Probably Safe	
Mestranol Norinyl, Ortho-Novum, Nelova, Ortho-Novum	• Female Sex Hormone	Probably Safe when used in the 'pill'	
Metformin Glucophage, Apo-Metformin, Rhoxal-Metformin	• Type 2 (adult) Diabetes Mellitus • Polycystic Ovaries	Possibly Safe	
Methadone Dolophine, Metadol, Opioids	• Opioid Dependence	Probably Safe	The baby may experience a withdrawal syndrome.

DRUG NAME	COMMON USE	FETAL SAFETY	REMARKS
Methicillin	• Antibiotic	Safe	
Methimazole Thiamazole, Tapazole	• Hyperthyroidism	**UNSAFE**	May cause malformations of skin; the drug of choice in pregnancy is propylthiouracil.
Methotrexate Rheumatrex	• Cancer • Arthritis • Autoimmune Diseases	**UNSAFE**	Can cause congenital malformations.
Methoxsalen Oxsoralen, Oxsoralen-Ultra, Ultramop	• Psoriasis	Unknown	
Methyldopa Aldoclor, Aldomet, Aldoril, Apo-Methyldopa, Nu-Medopa	• Hypertension	Safe	
Methylphenidate (HCL) Ritalin, Ritalin-SR	• Attention Deficit Disorder	Unknown	
Metoclopramide Apo-Metoclop, Metoclopramide Omega, Nu-Metoclopramide	• Vomiting	Probably Safe	
Metoprolol Succinate: Toprol-XL; Tartrate: Lopressor, Betabloc, Durules, Novo-Metoprolol, Apo-Metoprolol	• Hypertension	Possibly Safe	
Metronidazole Flagyl, Florazole ER, Noritate, NidaGel, Metro Cream/Gel; Combination Form: Metronidazole/Nystatin	• Trichomonal Infection Ulcer Disease	Probably Safe	

DRUG NAME	COMMON USE	FETAL SAFETY	REMARKS
Mexiletine Mexitil, Novo-Mexiletine	• Heartbeat Irregularities	Possibly Safe	
Miconazole Micatin, Micozole, Monistat Derm Cream/Vagcream	• Fungal Infections	Possibly Safe	
Midazolam (belongs to the Valium group) Versed	• Sedation for Surgery	Possibly Safe	Possible risk of oral clefts.
Mifeprex Mifepristone RU 486	• Pregnancy Termination	Unknown	Causes malformations in animals.
Minocycline	• Antibiotic	**UNSAFE**	May accumulate in baby's teeth after 8 weeks of pregnancy.
Minoxidil Loniten, Rogaine, Apo-Gain	• Hypertension	Unknown	
Mirtazapine Remeron	• Depression	Possibly Safe	
Misoprostol Cytotec, Combination Form: Arthrotec	• Peptic Ulcer • Gastric Acidity	**UNSAFE**	Causes the Moebius syndrome (facial paralysis with other malformation).
Moexipril	• Hypertension	**UNSAFE**	May cause renal shutdown and death in baby; should be switched to another antihypertensive drug.
Montelukast Singulair	• Asthma	Possibly Safe	
Morphine HP Sulfate: Kadian, MS Contin, Statex, Astramorph, Duramorph, MS Contin, MSIR Tablets, Oramorph SR, Rescudose, Roxanol, HCL: Opioids	• Pain	Probably Safe	When used near term, the baby may suffer withdrawal.

DRUG NAME	COMMON USE	FETAL SAFETY	REMARKS
Nadolol Corgard, Novo-Nadolol, Apo-Nadol	• Hypertension	Probably Safe	May cause intrauterine growth retardation.
Nafcillin Unipen	• Antibiotic	Safe	
Nalidixic Acid NegGram	• Antibiotic	Possibly Safe	
Naloxone Narcan, Talwin Nx	• Reversing Opioid Overdose	Possibly Safe	
Naproxen Naprosyn, Aleve, Anaprox, Aflaxen	• Pain • Inflammation	Probably Safe	May cause premature closure of the fetal vessel (ductus arteriosus).
Naratriptan Amerge	• Migraine Headaches	Unknown	
Nedocromil Sodium Tilade	• Asthma Prevention	Probably Safe	
Nefazodone Serzone-5HT, Lin-Nefazodone, Apo-Nefazodone	• Depression	Probably Safe	
Nelfinavir Viracept	• HIV1 Infections causing AIDs	Possibly Safe	Important to treat pregnant HIV-positive women to prevent morbidity and neonatal infection.
Neomycin Neosporin, Maxitrol, Kenacomb, Cortisporin, Ratio-Triacomb, Cortimyxin	• Antibiotic	Possibly Safe	
Nevirapine Viramune	• HIV1 Infections causing AIDs	Possibly Safe	Important to treat pregnant HIV-positive women to prevent morbidity and neonatal infection.
Nicardipine Cardene, Cardene SR	• Hypertension	Possibly Safe	

DRUG NAME	COMMON USE	FETAL SAFETY	REMARKS
Nifedipine Adalat, Adalat XL, Calcium Channel Blockers, Procardia	• Hypertension	Possibly Safe	
Nisoldipine Sular	• Hypertension	Possibly Safe	
Nitrofurantoin Macrodantin, MacroBID	• Urinary Infection	Probably Safe	
Nitroglycerin Minitran, Nitrates, Nitro-Dur, Nitrol, Nitrolingual Pumpspray, Nitrostat, Transderm-Nitro, Deponit, Nitrodisc	• Dilatation of Arteries	Probably Safe	
Nonoxynol Advantage 24	• Spermicide	Safe	
Norepinephrine Levophed	• Shock	Possibly Safe	
Norethindrone Micronor, Norlutate, Brevicon, Tri-Norinyl, Norinyl, Ovcon, Nelova; Combination Form: Estalis-Sequi, Estracomb, FemHRT, Loestrin, Minestrin, Synphasic, Ortho-Novum, Novo-Norfloxacin	• Female Sex Hormone	Probably Safe when used in 'pill'	
Norethynodrel	• Female Sex Hormone	Probably Safe when used in 'pill'	
Norfloxacin Novo-Norfloxacin, Noroxin, Apo-Norflaxin, Chibroxin	• Antibiotic	Probably Safe	

DRUG NAME	COMMON USE	FETAL SAFETY	REMARKS
Nortriptyline Pamelor	• Depression	Probably Safe	
Ofloxacin Floxin, Ocuflox	• Antibiotic	Probably Safe	
Olsalazine Dipentum	• Inflammatory Bowel Disease	Probably Safe	
Omeprazole Prilosec Delayed-Release	• Peptic Ulcer • Hyperactivity	Probably Safe	
Ondansetron HCL Zofran	• Vomiting	Probably Safe	
Oral Contraceptives Levogesternel, Norethindrone, Norgestimate, Norgestrel	• Pregnancy Prevention	Probably Safe when used appropriately	
Orlistat Xenical	• Obesity	Possibly Safe	
Oxacillin Sodium	• Antibiotic	Safe	
Oxcarbazepine Trileptal	• Epileptic Seizures	Possibly Safe	
Oxycodone Percodan; Combination Form: Opioids, Oxy-IR, Oxy-Contin, Endocet, Percocet, Endodan, Percodan, Percodan-Demi	• Pain	Possibly Safe	When used near term, the baby may suffer withdrawal.
Oxymetazoline (HCL) Nasal Spray, Long Lasting Nasal Spray, Claritin Allergic Congestion Relief	• Nasal Congestion	Probably Safe when used locally as recommended	
Pancuronium Pavulon	• Relaxation in Surgery	Probably Safe	

DRUG NAME	COMMON USE	FETAL SAFETY	REMARKS
Pantoprazole Panto IV, Pantoloc	• Peptic Ulcer • Gastric Acidity	Probably Safe	
Paroxetine Paxil	• Depression	Probably Safe	When used to term, baby may experience withdrawal.
Penicillamine Cuprimine, Depen Titratable	• Wilson's Disease	**UNSAFE**	May cause neonatal skin disorder (cutis loxa).
Penicillin Bicillin	• Antibiotic	Safe	
Pentamidine Pentacarinat, Nebupent, Pentam	• Pneumocystic Carinii Infection	Possibly Safe	
Pentoxifylline Trental	• Blood Clotting Prevention	Possibly Safe	
Permethrin Nix Cream Rinse, Elimite, Rid Lice Control Spray, Dermal Cream	• Scarbies Topical Treatment	Probably Safe	
Perphenazine Trilafon, Triavil	• Schizophrenia • Vomiting	Probably Safe	
Phenobarbital Arco-Lase Plus Tablets, Bellatal, Donnatal, Barbiturates, Phenobarbitone	• Sleeplessness • Anxiety • Epileptic Seizures	**UNSAFE**	May cause congenital malformations; when used near term, baby may experience withdrawal.
Phenylbutazone Apo-Phenylbutazone	• Pain • Inflammation	Unknown	

DRUG NAME	COMMON USE	FETAL SAFETY	REMARKS
Phenylephrine Atrohist, Ricobid, Comtrex, Dimetane-DC, Exgest LA, Propagest, Sinulin, Triaminic, Despec Caplets, Dura-Gest; Combination Form: Dristan, Dimetapp Nighttime Cold, Hycomine, Novahis-trex DH, Diphenyl-T, Zincfrin	• Shock • Allergic Reaction to Eyes and Ears (local use)	Unclear	
Phenylpropanolamine HCL Combination Form: Poly-Histine, Vanex Forte	• Appetite Control • Symptoms of Upper Respiratory Tract Infection and Allergy	Unclear	
Phenytoin Dilantin	• Epileptic Seizures	**UNSAFE**	May cause malformations of brain, face, and fingers.
Pindolol Visken, Viskazide	• Hypertension	Possibly Safe	
Pioglitazone Actos	• Type 2 (adult) Diabetes Mellitus	Unclear	
Piperazine Estropipate	• Worm Infection	Possibly Safe	
Piperacillin Pipracil, Tazocin	• Antibiotic	Safe	
Piroxicam Feldene, Nu-Pirox	• Pain • Inflammation	Possibly Safe	When used near term, may cause closure of the fetal vessel (ductus arteriosus).
Potassium Iodide	• Cough	**UNSAFE**	Contains iodine, which may adversely affect fetal thyroid development.

DRUG NAME	COMMON USE	FETAL SAFETY	REMARKS
Pravastatin Pravachol	• High Cholesterol	Unclear	
Praziquantel Biltricide	• Worm Infection	Unknown	
Prednisone Inflammation	• Asthma • Autoimmune Condition	Possibly Safe	May increase risk of cleft palate and lip in first trimester; may help mature fetal lungs, prevent prematurity.
Primidone Primaclone, Mysoline	• Epileptic Seizures	**UNSAFE**	May cause congenital malformation; when used near term, the baby may experience withdrawal.
Procainamide Procan SR, Pronestyl-SR	• Irregular Heartbeat	Possibly Safe	Has been used to treat fetal irregularities in heart beat.
Procarbazine Matulane	• Cancer	**UNSAFE**	Can cause congenital malformations; most risk in first trimester.
Prochlorperazine Compazine; Combination Form: Nu-Prochlor, Stemetil, Apo-Prochlorazine	• Psychosis • Vomiting	Probably Safe	
Promethazine HCL Phenergan, Mepergan	• Antihistamine	Probably Safe	
Propofol Diprivan	• Anesthesia for Surgery • Sedation	Possibly Safe	
Propranolol Inderal-LA, Nu-Propranolol	• Hypertension	Probably Safe	May cause fetal growth restriction.
Propylthiouracil Paladin	• Hyperthyroidism	Possibly Safe	May affect fetal thyroid at high dose.

DRUG NAME	COMMON USE	FETAL SAFETY	REMARKS
Pseudoephedrine Pseudofrin, Sudafed Decongestant, Eltor; Combination Form: Dimetapp Daytime Cold, Dristan N.D., Sinutab Sinus, Tylenol Sinus, Sinutab Sinus and Allergy, Tylenol Cold, Sinutab with Codeine, Triaminic Cold, Robitussin Honey Flu, Balminil Cough & Flu, Benylin 4 Flu, Tylenol Flu, CoA\ctified Tablets, Robitussin Cough & Cold, Advil Cold and Sinus, Sudafed Sinus Advance, Trinalin, Claritin Extra	• Allergy • Nasal Congestion • Upper Respiratory Tract Infection	Possibly Safe	
Pyridostigmine Mestinon, Mestinon-SR, Regonol	• Myasthenia Gravis	Possibly Safe	
Quinapril Accupril, Accuretic, ACE Inhibitors	• Hypertension	**UNSAFE**	May cause renal shutdown and death in baby; should be switched to another drug.
Quinidine Biquin Durules, Apo-Quinidine	• Irregular Heart Beat	Possibly Safe	
Quinine Quinamm	• Malaria	Possibly Safe	
Ramipril Altace	• Hypertension	**UNSAFE**	May cause renal shutdown, skull anomalies, and death; should be switched to another drug.
Ranitidine Zantac	• Peptic Ulcer • Gastric Acidity	Probably Safe	

DRUG NAME	COMMON USE	FETAL SAFETY	REMARKS
Repaglinide Gluconorm	• Type 2 (adult) Diabetes Mellitus	Unclear	
Rifampin Combination Form: Rifampicin, Rifadin, Rifampin, Rofact, Rifater	• Tuberculosis	Possibly Safe	
Ritodrine HCL Yutopar	• Premature Uterine Contractions	Probably Safe	
Ritonavir Combination Form: Norvir, Norvir Sec, Kaletra	• HIV1 Infections causing AIDs	Possibly Safe	It is important to treat HIV to ensure maternal health and prevent
Rizatriptan Maxalt, Maxalt PRD	• Migraine Headache	Unknown	
Rofecoxib Vioxx	• Pain • Inflammation	Unknown	
Rosiglitazone Avandia	• Type 2 (adult) Diabetes Mellitus	Unknown	
Saquinavir Fortovase Roche, Invirase	• HIV1 Infections causing AIDs	Possibly Safe	It is important to treat HIV to ensure maternal health and prevent neonatal infection.
Sertraline Zoloft	• Depression	Probably Safe	
Simvastatin Zocor	• High Cholesterol	Unknown	
Sotalol Nu-Sotalol, Sotacor, Betapace	• Heartbeat Irregularities	Possibly Safe	
Sparfloxacin	• Antibiotic	Possibly Safe	
Spiramycin Rovamycine	• Toxoplasmosis	Probably Safe	

DRUG NAME	COMMON USE	FETAL SAFETY	REMARKS
Spironolactone Aldactone; Combination Form: Aldactazide, Novo-Spirozide	• Water Retention	Unknown	
Stavudine D4T, Zerit	• HIV1 Infections causing AIDs	Possibly Safe	It is important to treat HIV to ensure maternal health and prevent neonatal infection.
Streptokinase Kabikinase	• Blood Clotting	Probably Safe	
Sufentanil Sufenta, Opioids	• Pain • Anesthesia for Surgery	Probably Safe	When used near term, baby may experience withdrawal.
Sulfasalazine Salazopyrin, Salazopyrin En-Tabs, Azulfidine	• Inflammatory Bowel Disease	Probably Safe	
Sulfonamides Trimazine, Co Trimazole, Septra, Bactrim	• Anti-infective	Probably Safe	May decrease folate levels and increase risk of certain malformations.
Sulindac Apo-Sulin, Clinoril	• Pain • Inflammation	Probably Safe	When used near term, may close the fetal vessel (ductus arteriosus).
Sumatriptan Imitrex Nasal Spray, Imitrex	• Migraine Headache	Probably Safe	
Tacrolimus Prograf, Protopic	• Organ Transplant	Possibly Safe	
Tamoxifen Tamofen, Nolvadex, Nolvadex-D, Apo-Tamox	• Cancer	Unknown	
Terbutaline Bricanyl Turbuhaler, Brethaire Inhaler, Bricanyl Injection	• Asthma	Probably Safe	

DRUG NAME	COMMON USE	FETAL SAFETY	REMARKS
Terfenadine Seldane, Seldane-D	• Allergy	Probably Safe	
Tetracycline Achromycin, Topicycline, Apo-Tetra, Novo-Tetra, Nu-Tetra	• Antibiotic	**UNSAFE**	May adversely affect fetal teeth after 8 weeks of pregnancy.
Thalidomide Contergan, Distaval	• Leprosy • HIV • Organ Transplant	**UNSAFE**	Limb malformation and other internal organ malformations. Women on thalidomide must be protected against pregnancy.
Theophylline Thiamazole	• Asthma	Probably Safe	
Thioguanine Thioguanine Tablets	• Cancer	**UNSAFE**	Can cause major malformations; most risk in first trimester.
Ticarcillin Timentin, Ticar	• Antibiotic	Safe	
Timolol Apo-Timop, Gen-Timolol, Timoptic, Timoptic-XE; Combination Form: Cosopt, Timpilo	• Hypertension	Possibly Safe	
Tinzaparin Heparins, Innohep	• Blood Clotting	Safe	
Tobramycin Tobrex, Nebcin, TOBI, Tobradex	• Antibiotic	Possibly Safe	
Tolazamide Tolinase	• Type 2 (adult) Diabetes Mellitus	Possibly Safe	May cause neonatal hypoglycemia.
Tolbutamide APO-Tolbutamide, Sulfonylureas	• Type 2 (adult) Diabetes Mellitus	Possibly Safe	May cause neonatal hypoglycemia.

DRUG NAME	COMMON USE	FETAL SAFETY	REMARKS
Trazodone Desyrel	• Depression	Possibly Safe	
Tretinoin Retin-A	• Acne • Skin Disorders	Possibly Safe	
Triazolam Halcion, Apo-Triazo	• Sleeplessness	Possibly Safe	When used near term, the baby may experience withdrawal.
Trifluoperazine Apo-Trifluoperazine	• Psychosis • Vomiting	Probably Safe	
Trimethoprim Coptin, Proloprim	• Anti-infective	Probably Safe	
Tripelennamine PBZ, PBZ-SR	• Allergies	Probably Safe	
Triprolidine Actifed, Ratio-Cortidin	• Allergies	Probably Safe	
Trovafloxacin Alatrofloxacin	• Antibiotic	Unknown	
Urokinase Abbokinase	• Blood Clotting	Safe	
Valacyclovir Valtrex	• Herpes Infection	Possibly Safe	
Valproic Acid Depakene, Epiject I.V., Rhoxal-Valproic	• Epileptic Seizures • Psychiatric Conditions	**UNSAFE**	Increase risk of neural tube defects. Other malformations suspected but not proven.
Valsartan Diovan	• Hypertension	**UNSAFE**	May theoretically cause neonatal renal shutdown and neonatal death; should be switched to another anti-hypertensive drug
Vancomycin Vancocin, Vancoled	• Antibiotic	Safe	

DRUG NAME	COMMON USE	FETAL SAFETY	REMARKS
Venlafaxine Effexor	• Depression	Probably Safe	
Verapamil Calan SR, Isoptin	• Heart Rate Irregularities	Possibly Safe	
Vinblastine Oncovin	• Cancer	**UNSAFE**	Can cause malformations; most risk in first trimester.
Vincristine Oncovin	• Cancer	**UNSAFE**	Can cause malformations; most risk in first trimester.
Zalcitabine Hivid	• HIV1 Infections causing AIDs	Possibly Safe	It is important to treat HIV to ensure maternal health and prevent neonatal infection.
Zidovudine Retrovir	• HIV1 Infections causing AIDs	Probably Safe	It is important to treat HIV to ensure maternal health and prevent neonatal infection.

RESOURCES

Koren G, ed. Maternal-Fetal Toxicology. A Clinician's Guide. 3rd ed. New York: Marcel Dekker, 2001.

Visit the Motherisk website at www.motherisk.org and click on "Drugs in Pregnancy." Then find the category of drug that you wish to read more about (for example, "Antihistamines") and follow the links to the references and abstracts. The 'What's New' box on the website's main page links visitors to Motherisk's latest research findings.

CHAPTER SEVEN

Over-the-Counter Medications

Q. *I have just found out I am pregnant. This is allergy season, and I don't think I can function at work without antihistamines. How safe are antihistamines during pregnancy?*

— *Motherisk Caller*

A. *Based on a large number of studies, antihistamines do not increase risk for fetal malformations. During early pregnancy, a critical stage of organogenesis that might be adversely affected by drugs and environmental agents, women receive more prescriptions for antihistamines than for any other agent except vitamins. Antihistamines are used during early pregnancy mainly to treat morning sickness.*

— *Motherisk Counselor*

There are thousands of over-the-counter medications. Adults use them to treat everything from coughs and colds to heartburn and skin irritations. However, one of the Ten Commandments for a Safe and Healthy Pregnancy states, *Do Not Self-Prescribe.* The reason is simple: some medications that are safe before pregnancy may not be safe for the fetus.

Although we cannot provide a safety and risk assessment for every available over-the-counter medication, we can offer an evaluation of some of the more common groups. Brand names are used occasionally to help you identify certain medications. We are not, however, endorsing one brand over another.

RISK GRADES

At Motherisk, we have established a system for grading the risk of prescription and over-the-counter drugs in pregnancy, ranging from 'Safe' to 'Unsafe'. This does not mean that everything that is not deemed 'Safe' is 'Unsafe' and must be avoided during pregnancy. There are *degrees of safety* that should be considered, especially if the medication is important for the health and well-being of the mother. These degrees of safety are vital to balancing the benefit and the risk of various medications.

Safe

Safe means that a convincing and authoritative body of scientific evidence, accumulated over time, through sound scientific research, shows no adverse effects on the fetus.

Probably Safe

Probably Safe means that there is no evidence the drug is dangerous to the fetus and that the information showing it to be safe is rather large. Here, the benefit/risk assessment will be weighted, in most cases, in favor of using the medication.

Possibly Safe

Possibly Safe means that there is no evidence that the drug is dangerous for the fetus, but the information showing it to be safe is limited. By 'limited' we mean that only a few studies have been published in the medical literature, or the studies that are available do not meet all of the rigorous standards of critical scientific appraisal.

Unsafe

Unsafe means that there is evidence to show that the medication may cause harmful effects during pregnancy or during a particular trimester of pregnancy. This does not mean that the harm is certain to happen in each and every case of exposure, but there is enough risk of harm to justify careful use or avoidance in pregnancy.

Unknown or Unclear

Unknown or *Unclear* means that there is simply not enough reliable information for us to be able to determine safety or risk in pregnancy. This may change over time as evidence-based research uncovers more information about the effects of these drugs.

LOOK BACK

Consult the *Guide to Safety/Risk of Prescription Drugs in Pregnancy* in Chapter 6 when evaluating any over-the-counter drugs medications you are taking or considering taking since some of the OTC ingredients may be described in that Guide. Our determination of risk or safety is based upon the same criteria that we applied to prescription drugs in Chapter 6.

Treating Common Health Conditions

If you use a medication that is not mentioned in the following FAQs, you may wish to contact a teratogen information service near you. Their contact numbers are listed in the "Resources" section. Often a medication is a mixture of two or more active ingredients, so it will be important to check out all ingredients. And again, please remember that the information we provide here is not meant to replace the advice of your doctor or other health-care providers. Consult them before using any over-the-counter medication.

Acne

Q *Before I got pregnant, I used a retinol cream for acne. Can I continue to use it now that I'm pregnant?*

A Retinol is not a 'drug of choice' in pregnancy because it contains vitamin A. High amounts of vitamin A (more than 50,000 IU) can cause birth defects and should be avoided during pregnancy. That's why prescription acne drugs, such as isotretinoin (Accutane), should not be used during pregnancy. In fact, Accutane is so highly teratogenic that a woman who wants to use it must sign a document stating that she will use two forms of contraception to prevent pregnancy during the time that she is on this prescription medication.

Allergies

Q *It's allergy season again and my hay fever is driving me crazy. What's safe for me now that I'm pregnant?*

A The most widely used medications for allergies are the 'old' (or sedating) antihistamines. There are scores of these available over the counter. They have been shown by numerous large studies not to increase fetal risk.

SAFETY/RISK
Drugs of Choice

Though retinol has not been shown to increase risk to the fetus, your safest choice is not to use it while you are pregnant. The drugs of choice for the treatment of acne during pregnancy are topical erythromycin, clindamycin, and benzoyl peroxide. You should talk to your doctor in order to make the best choice.

However, most people now use the newer, non-sedating antihistamines to treat seasonal allergies. These drugs are *probably safe* (based on several studies), although the amount of evidence in favor of their use is much smaller than what supports the fetal safety of the old, sedating antihistamines.

Motherisk conducted a meta-analysis of all controlled studies of antihistamine use in early pregnancy, in order to quantify the relative risk of major malformations associated with antihistamine use. Twenty-four studies met our inclusion criteria; more than 200,000 women were involved. Our analysis indicated no positive association between the use of antihistamines in the first trimester and rates of major malformations.

Colds

Q Everyone in my family has been sniffling and sneezing for days. Now I've caught their cold and I'm pregnant. Is there something I can take?

A Cold remedies typically contain several ingredients, including analgesic antipyretics (to decrease body temperature and to treat aches and pains), antihistamines (to dry the nasal cavity and eyes), and decongestants (to decrease congestion of the nose). In general, the analgesic antipyretics may include acetaminophen. Acetaminophen is *safe* for the fetus.

The 'old' antihistamines that make you sleepy, such as chlorpheniramine (Chlor Tripolon) and diphenhydramine (Benadryl), are generally safe. In fact, sedating antihistamines, such as dimenhydrinate, are widely used to prevent nausea and vomiting in pregnancy (morning sickness).

Anticongestants contained in cold remedies are typically sympathomimetic medications (those that act on sympathetic nerves). They usually include noradrenaline, ephedrine, and phenylpropanolamine. Noradrenaline and ephedrine are *probably safe* in small, infrequent amounts. Phenylpropanolamine has been associated with a rare malformation of the abdominal wall of the fetus called gastroschisis. It also may cause vascular events in adults, and has been recently removed from cold remedies.

SAFETY/RISK

Avoid ASA and NSAIDs

ASA (acetylsalicylic acid, such as aspirin) and other non-steroidal anti-inflammatory drugs (NSAIDs), such as ibuprofen and naproxen, should be avoided in late pregnancy (the last 3 months). The concern with NSAIDs is that they may prematurely close the ductus arteriosus, a fetal blood vessel that normally causes blood to bypass the fetal lungs directly into the aorta.

Constipation

Q *I'm trying to eat 'healthy' with plenty of fiber in my diet, but there are still days when constipation is a problem. I'd like to take something for it but what are my options?*

A For constipation it is best to eat high fiber (e.g., bran) cereal. If your health-care providers believe you need medication, they will likely recommend agents such as psyllium mucilloid (e.g., Metamucil) and fibyrax to facilitate bulk formation.

Cough

Q *The sniffles are gone, but I've still got the cough that came with this cold. Is there anything I can take?*

A Cough lozenges and expectorants, such as guaifenesin (Robitussin plain), to reduce phlegm are *probably safe*. Cough suppressants, such as dextromethorphan, are also *probably safe* when used for a short time.

Heartburn

Q *I'm 6 months pregnant and getting occasional bouts of heartburn. Is there something I can take to relieve the symptoms?*

A Pregnancy is characterized by an increase in the rate and severity of heartburn. As a first step to relieving heartburn symptoms, try making changes in your diet. If that doesn't work, speak to your health-care provider about treatment. Most preparations for heartburn include antacids to neutralize acids. Aluminum hydroxide and magnesium hydroxide (Maalox) or alginic compound (Gaviscon) are *safe*. Calcium carbonate, such as Tums and Rolaids, are also *safe*.

Some products include medications such as H2 blockers (e.g., ranitidine) that decrease the production of acids. These medications are *probably safe* in pregnancy.

Avoid antacids with sodium or salicylates (Pepto Bismol) because the sodium load may not be healthy for you.

SAFETY/RISK

Stool Softeners

Stool softeners, such as docusate sodium (e.g., Colace), calcium glycerin, sorbitol, and lactulose, are probably safe in pregnancy. Avoid gastrointestinal stimulants, such as bisacodyl.

Pain Killers

Q I usually take acetaminophen for occasional headache pain. Can I continue to do that now that I'm pregnant?

A The most commonly used painkillers include acetaminophen, which is safe for the fetus. The non-steroidal anti-inflammatory drugs (NSAIDs) are probably safe during the first trimester of pregnancy, but in late pregnancy may cause closure of the fetal ductus arteriosus. See our discussion of "Cold Remedies" above.

> **SAFETY/RISK**
>
> **4th Commandment**
> Remember the 4th Commandment:
> Do not self-prescribe.
> Speak to your doctor or other health-care provider before taking any over-the-counter medications.

Sleep Disturbance

Q I'm usually a good sleeper but some of the discomforts of pregnancy are beginning to affect my sleep. Is there something I can take?

A While some women may need prescription drugs (e.g., benzodiazopine), occasional sleep disturbance during pregnancy can be effectively and safely treated with sedating antihistamines, such as diphenhydramine and doxylamine.

Skin Irritation (Itching)

Q My doctor has assured me that it's nothing serious — just a rash — but still the itching is bothersome. Is there something I can take or must I stick to topical treatments only?

A Moisturizing creams and lotions, Aveeno oatmeal bath, zinc oxide cream or ointment, and calamine lotion are all *safe* topical treatments. The most widely used and safe oral medication is hydroxyzine (Atarax).

CHAPTER EIGHT

Herbal Products and Natural Medicines

Q. *I'm 9 weeks pregnant and have been doing fine, but I'm a bit concerned that I might be coming down with a cold (everyone else in the house is sneezing!). I always talk to my doctor before I take any medications, but I'm assuming that I don't need to consult her about herbal products that I used regularly before I got pregnant. Is that right?*

— Motherisk Caller

A. *No. Speak to your doctor first. Just because it's 'herbal' doesn't mean it is safe for use in pregnancy.*

— Motherisk Counselor

More and more women of childbearing age are using herbal products and natural medicines. Part of their appeal is a general notion that 'herbal' or 'natural' means safe. Unfortunately, this naive approach to herbal products overlooks the fact that some very potent and strictly regulated drugs for illnesses, such as cancer and heart disease, are produced from plants. Of course, no responsible pharmacist would ever think of dispensing these potent plant-derived medications without a prescription. Yet many consumers buy and use unregulated herbal medicines for all sorts of conditions without proper guidance.

RISK GRADES

At Motherisk, we have established a system for grading the risk of prescription and over-the-counter drugs in pregnancy, ranging from 'Safe' to 'Unsafe'. This does not mean that everything that is not deemed 'Safe' is 'Unsafe' and must be avoided during pregnancy. There are *degrees of safety* that should be considered, especially if the medication is important for the health and well-being of the mother. These degrees of safety are vital to balancing the benefit and the risk of various medications.

Safe

Safe means that a convincing and authoritative body of scientific evidence, accumulated over time, through sound scientific research, shows no adverse effects on the fetus.

Probably Safe

Probably Safe means that there is no evidence the drug is dangerous to the fetus and that the information showing it to be safe is rather large. Here, the benefit/risk assessment will be weighted, in most cases, in favor of using the medication.

Possibly Safe

Possibly Safe means that there is no evidence that the drug is dangerous for the fetus, but the information showing it to be safe is limited. By 'limited' we mean that only a few studies have been published in the medical literature, or the studies that are available do not meet all of the rigorous standards of critical scientific appraisal.

Unsafe

Unsafe means that there is evidence to show that the medication may cause harmful effects during pregnancy or during a particular trimester of pregnancy. This does not mean that the harm is certain to happen in each and every case of exposure, but there is enough risk of harm to justify careful use or avoidance in pregnancy.

Unknown or Unclear

Unknown or *Unclear* means that there is simply not enough reliable information for us to be able to determine safety or risk in pregnancy. This may change over time as evidence-based research uncovers more information about the effects of these drugs.

Lack of Regulation

Unlike prescription drugs, herbal products are not labeled as 'drugs' but rather as foods by regulatory agencies like the Federal Drug Administration (FDA) in the United States and the Natural Health Products Directorate (NHPD) in Canada and have not been widely tested for either safety or effectiveness until recently. Because the industry is not highly regulated, the chemical content of different brands of the same herbal products made by different manufacturers may have very different levels of the active ingredients.

For most of these products, there is little or no information about their safety in pregnancy. The Motherisk Program is trying to fill the information gap by systematically following up pregnancy outcome in women who have taken natural products. So far, we have established the relative safety of echinacea and ginger. We are now collecting data on St. John's wort, but it will be some time before the results are in. In the meantime, pregnant women and women planning pregnancy should proceed with caution.

Guide to Safety/Risk of Herbal Products and Natural Medicines in Pregnancy

NOTES ON USING THIS CHART

Abortifacient and Emmenagogue

Two other terms are especially important when assessing herbal products. Abortifacient means that the substance induces abortion. Emmenagogue means that the substance induces uterine bleeding. Clearly, both abortifacients and emmenagogues should be avoided during pregnancy.

Common Use

By "common use" we mean the most frequent application of the product as reported in the medical literature. We are not convinced that these products necessarily work for the indication shown and do not endorse or recommend their use.

Nomenclature

For each herb, the common name is given first, followed by its botanical name and family (in parentheses). Synonyms then follow.

HERBAL NAME	COMMON USE	FETAL SAFETY	REMARKS
Alfalfa *Medicago sativa* L. (Fabaceae)	• High Cholesterol • Menopause	Probably Safe when used as food	Restrict to dietary use.
Aloe Vera *Aloe Vera* (L.) Burm. f. (Aloeaceae)	• Infections • Inflammation • Laxative	**UNSAFE**	Induces abortions in animals.
Black Cohosh *Cimicifuga racemosa* (L.) Nutt. (Ranunculaceae) Black Snakeroot, Rattleweed	• Premenstrual Syndrome • Dysmenorrhea • Menopause	**UNSAFE**	Binds to estrogen receptors. Used to induce uterine contraction. There are cases of uncontrolled contraction with fetal distress.
Burdock *Arctium lappa* L. (Asteraceae) Beggar's Button, Burr Seed, Clotbur, Cocklebur, Hardock, Turkey Burseed, Cress	• Water Retention • Constipation • Fever • Infections	**UNSAFE**	May stimulate uterine contraction.
Calendula *Calendula officinalis* L. (Asteraceae) Pot Marigold, Mary Bud	• Gastritis • Ulcers	**UNSAFE**	Orally, may be an emmenagogue.
Capsicum *Capsicum annuum* L. (Solanaceae) Cayenne Pepper, Red Pepper, Chili Pepper, Bird Pepper	• Pain	Safe when used as food only at dietary doses	Restrict to dietary use only. In high doses, this agent may stimulate uterine contractions.
Chamomile *Matricaria recutita* L. (Asteraceae)	• Gastrointestinal Discomfort • Sleeplessness • Anxiety	**UNSAFE**	Was used traditionally to induce abortion.
Cascara Sagrada *Rhamnus purshianus* (Rhamnaceae)	• Constipation	Possibly Safe	This is a *stimulant* laxative and as such is not the best choice for use in pregnancy. Safer choices are bulk forming agents or stool softeners.

HERBAL NAME	COMMON USE	FETAL SAFETY	REMARKS
Chaste Tree *Vitex agnus-castus* L. (Verbenaceae)	• Premenstrual Syndrome • Menopause • Insufficient Lactation	**UNSAFE**	This is an emmenagogue.
Cranberry *Vaccinium macrocarpon* Ait. (Ericaceae)	• Urinary Tract Infection	Safe when used as food	Restrict to dietary use.
Dandelion Root *Taraxacum officinale* G.H. Weber ex Wiggers (Asteraceae)	• Liver-Bile Conditions • Dyspepsia • Lack of Appetite • Leaves: Water Retention	Probably Safe in low dose	
Devil's Claw *Harpagophytum procumbens* DC. (Pedaliaceae)	• Joint Inflammation • Indigestion	Unknown/ Unclear	
Dong Quai *Angelica sinensis* (Oliv.) Diels (Apiaceae) Chinese Angelica	• Menopause • Dysmenorrhea • Amenorrhea	**UNSAFE**	Considered traditional emmenagogue and abortifacient.
Echinacea *E. angustifolia, E. purpurea, E. pallida* (Asteraceae) Purple Coneflower	• Upper Respiratory Tract Infections	Probably Safe	
Evening Primrose *Oenothera biennis* L. (Onagraceae)	• Atopic Eczema • Premenstrual Syndrome • Menopause • Endometritis • Psychiatric Conditions	Probably Safe	Less than 4 g/day.
Feverfew *Tanacetum parthenium* (L.) Schultz-Bip. (Asteraceae) Chrysanthemum, Midsummer Daisy	• Migraine Prevention	**UNSAFE**	Traditional emmenogogue and abortifacient.

HERBAL NAME	COMMON USE	FETAL SAFETY	REMARKS
Garlic *Allium sativum* L. (Lilliaceae)	• Infections • High Lipids	Probably Safe	
Ginger *Zingiber officinale* Roscoe (Zingiberaceae)	• Nausea and Vomiting	Probably Safe	
Ginkgo *Ginkgo biloba* L. (Ginkgoaceae)	• Dementia • Memory Impairment	Unknown/ Unclear	
Goldenseal *Hydrastis canadensis* L. (Ranunculaceae)	• Upper Respiratory Infection • Urinary Infection	**UNSAFE**	Causes uterine contractions.
Hops *Humulus lupulus* L. (Cannabaceae)	• Sleeplessness • Agitation • Dyspepsia • Irritable Bowel Syndrome	**UNSAFE**	Has hormone substances; relaxes uterine wall in experiments.
Juniper *Juniperus communis* L. (Cupressaceae)	• Urine Infections • Joint Inflammation • Indigestion	**UNSAFE**	Traditional emmenagogue and abortifacient.
Kava *Piper methysticum* G. Forst (Piperaceae) Kava-Kava	• Anxiety • Headache	Unknown/ Unclear	
Licorice *Glycyrrhiza glabra* L. (Fabaceae)	• Ulcers of the Gastric-Duodenal • Mouth Herpes • Canker Sores	**UNSAFE**	Traditional emmenogogue and abortifacient.
Ma Huang *Ephedra sinica* Stapf. (Ephredraceae) Ephedra	• Weight Loss • Asthma	**UNSAFE**	Ephedrine may stimulate the uterus.
Passionflower *Passiflor incarnata* L. (Passifloraceae)	• Sleeplessness • Tension • Restlessness	**UNSAFE**	Stimulates the uterus in animals.

HERBAL NAME	COMMON USE	FETAL SAFETY	REMARKS
Peppermint *Menta x piperita* L. (Lamiknaceae)	• Gastrointestinal Discomfort	**UNSAFE**	Traditional emmenagogue and arbortifacient.
Slippery Elm *Ulmus rubra* Muhl. (Ulmaceae)	• Orally: gastrointestinal ulcers, gastritis, cough • Topically: wound healing	**UNSAFE**	Traditional arbortifacient.
St. John's Wort *Hypericum perforatum* L. (Clusiaceae) Hypericum	• Depression	Probably Safe	
Tea Tree Oil *Melaleuco ulternifolia* (Maiden & Betche) *Cheel* (Myrtaceae)	• Fungal Infection	Unknown/ Unclear	
Uva-Ursi *Arctostaphylos uva-ursi* (L.) Spreng. (Ericaea) Bearberry	• Urinary Tract Infection	Unknown/ Unclear	
Valerian *Valerian officinalis* L. (Valerianaceae) Belgian Valerian, Common Valerian, Fragrant Valerian, Garden Valerian	• Sleeplessness • Anxiety • Restlessness	Possibly Safe	

Treating Depression with St. John's Wort

Q *I'm 23 years old, and I have been taking St. John's wort for postpartum depression for about two years. I am now planning my second pregnancy. Am I or my fetus at risk if I continue to take the herbal therapy?*

A Despite the widespread availability and use of St. John's wort and extensive research on the herb, there are almost no data on reproductive safety. At this stage, therefore, St. John's wort cannot be recommended as safe therapy during pregnancy.

In-Depth

St. John's wort (*Hypericum perforatum*) is the most common herbal therapy used for depression. In Germany, it accounted for one quarter of all antidepressant prescriptions in 1997. In North America, St. John's wort is a dietary supplement; in 1998, retail sales in the United States totaled $140 million. St. John's wort can be found at most pharmacies, natural food stores, and some grocery stores in North America and is widely available to women of childbearing age.

St. John's wort contains at least 10 different active substances; *hypericin* is considered the most active ingredient. The herbal extract acts like an antidepressant by inhibiting the synaptic absorption of serotonin, dopamine, and noradrenaline.

St. John's wort is well tolerated and is perceived as safer than most antidepressants prescribed. Responses from a randomly selected group of physicians, medical students, naturopaths, and naturopathic students to a detailed questionnaire (242 respondents; 38% response rate) showed that St. John's wort was the second most popular complementary medicine recommended by both medical doctors and naturopaths (echinacea was first). Although only one physician recommended a herbal product to a pregnant patient, as many as 49% of the naturopaths felt comfortable recommending herbal products to pregnant women.

However, St. John's wort can have adverse effects and interact with other drugs. About 2% to 26% of patients using St. John's wort report side effects that include nausea and restlessness (most common), delayed hypersensitivity, dizziness, dry mouth, and constipation. Photodermatitis (skin sensitivity to sun) is a rare, but well-recognized, adverse effect. St. John's wort may put transplant patients receiving cyclosporine at risk of graft rejection.

SAFETY/RISK ❖ Insufficient Studies

Whether recommended by a family physician or taken without recommendation, St. John's wort still has not been sufficiently studied to be declared safe in pregnancy. Much more preclinical and clinical data must be accumulated before the herb can safely be regulated as an adjunct or alternative treatment to the antidepressant drugs currently prescribed for pregnant women.

Animal Studies

Three animal studies have addressed use of St. John's wort during the perinatal period. No reproductive toxic effects were found in rats or dogs with oral doses of 900 and 2700 mg/kg. When a group of female mice receiving hypericum from 2 weeks before conception and throughout gestation was compared with a group of female mice receiving placebo, one study found that mouse offspring in both groups were similar in gestational age at delivery, litter size, perinatal outcome, body weight, body length, and head circumference growth through adulthood. Moreover, no differences were found in reaching physical milestones, in reproductive capability, or in growth and development of second-generation offspring. A similar study found lower birth weights among male offspring in the St. John's wort group, but no long-term differences in early developmental tasks, locomotor activity, or exploratory behavior throughout development.

Self-treatment

Only two cases of women treating themselves with St. John's wort during pregnancy are reported in the literature. In one case, where follow-up was available, a woman took the herb from 24 weeks gestation until delivery. Her neonate was reported to have normal results of physical examination and behavioral assessment during the first month of life.

Motherisk Study

Motherisk is currently conducting a prospective controlled study on St. John's wort during pregnancy and following up mothers who use the herb during lactation.

Using Echinacea for Colds

Q I commonly use herbal products; now I am planning a pregnancy. As we enter the 'cold and flu' season, I would like to know if the herb echinacea is safe in pregnancy.

A Although herbal products have been used in the past during pregnancy and delivery, there is little evidence showing they are safe. However, a recent Motherisk study showed that use of echinacea during the first trimester of pregnancy was not associated with increased risk of major malformations.

> **FACT** ✔
>
> **First Trimester Safety**
> Results of a major Motherisk study suggest that use of echinacea during the first trimester is not associated with increased risk for major malformations.

In-Depth

In 2000, Motherisk completed the first prospective controlled study addressing the safety of herbs during pregnancy using the herb echinacea. A total of 206 women who used echinacea products during pregnancy were enrolled into the study (112 used it during the first trimester). This cohort was disease-matched (upper respiratory tract ailments) to women exposed to nonteratogenic agents by maternal age and alcohol and cigarette use.

Aside from this recent study on use of echinacea, no other studies addressing safety during pregnancy have been completed.

RESOURCES

Koren G, ed. Maternal-Fetal Toxicology. A Clinician's Guide. 3rd ed. New York: Marcel Dekker, 2001: Chapter 31.

CHAPTER NINE

Alcohol, Smoking, and Drug Abuse

Q. I have been smoking since I was 13. I am now pregnant and I think I can kick the habit, but my friend says it is not good for the baby if I stop smoking cold turkey. Is she right?

— Motherisk Caller

A. Your friend is wrong. Smoking during pregnancy increases the risk of premature birth, stillbirth, and crib death (Sudden Infant Death Syndrome or SIDS).

— Motherisk Counselor

Alcohol

About one-half of all women in North America drink some alcohol as part of their normal life. About one-half of all pregnancies are unplanned. This means that around one-quarter of all babies born each year may be exposed to some alcohol before birth. That exposure is most likely to occur during early pregnancy.

SAFETY/RISK ❖ Refrain from Alcohol

Currently, it is not known how little alcohol it takes to cause damage to the baby. The best bet for women who are planning a pregnancy is to refrain from any drinking. Existing studies suggest, however, that the babies of non-problem drinkers, who were exposed to a few drinks in early pregnancy, before the women knew they had conceived, were normal. All cases of Fetal Alcohol Syndrome have been diagnosed among alcohol-dependent women.

Fetal Alcohol Syndrome

The most devastating result of problem-drinking during pregnancy is Fetal Alcohol Syndrome (FAS). FAS occurs in approximately 1 out of every 1,000 babies born. The full-blown syndrome includes problem maternal drinking, growth retardation (both during and after pregnancy), facial changes (including small eyes, a thin upper lip, an erased philtrum, the 'canal' that goes from the upper lip to the nose), and damage to the baby's brain.

However, for each full-blown case of Fetal Alcohol Syndrome, there are scores of babies who do not show these typical facial features. They are often described as having Fetal Alcohol Effects or Alcohol Related Neurodevelopment Disorder (ARND). Alcohol consumption during pregnancy can also cause Alcohol Related Birth Defects (ARBD) that affect the brain, heart, kidneys, liver, eyes, ears, and bones.

Fetal Alcohol Spectrum Disorder (FASD), a term introduced in 1999, acknowledges that alcohol consumption during pregnancy can cause a wide range of effects. Effects on brain development are the most devastating and may include cognitive effects (such as low IQ), language difficulties, learning disabilities, impulsivity, hyperactivity, severe problems in adaptability and in understanding social cues, and delinquency – to name just a few.

Since the first description of Fetal Alcohol Syndrome some 30 years ago, most women are aware that they should not drink during pregnancy, and, indeed, the number of drinkers in pregnancy has decreased substantially. Still, the number of alcohol-dependent women involved in problem drinking has not changed.

FREQUENTLY ASKED QUESTION

Q: My partner and I finally got away last month for a week of rest and relaxation. We really needed the break. Now I find that I'm pregnant and am very worried about the occasional drink we enjoyed during our week of fun in the sun. What should I do?

A: The Motherisk Alcohol and Substance Use Helpline gets frequent calls from women who describe this sort of inadvertent use of alcohol during pregnancy.

1. First, don't panic. Though there is no known safe level of alcohol exposure during pregnancy, there is little risk of fetal damage from an occasional drink consumed before you knew you were pregnant.

2. Second, now that you know you are pregnant, stop drinking alcohol. If you find that quitting is a challenge, then speak to your health-care provider or a teratogen counselor about where to go for help and support.

3. Third, educate yourself on the effects of alcohol during pregnancy and while breastfeeding so that you can better understand the risks.

LOOK AHEAD

See Chapter 14 for a means of calculating the time from beginning of drinking until clearance of alcohol from breast milk for women of various body weights.

Alcohol and Breastfeeding

After the birth of a child, many women wish to get back to their old lifestyle, which may include some drinking. Because alcohol crosses into the breast milk and it is not in the child's interest to be exposed to alcohol, mothers should either refrain from drinking while breastfeeding, or plan to drink in a way that will not allow alcohol to accumulate in the breast milk.

RESOURCES

The body of research on FASD is growing rapidly. The new on-line *Journal of FAS International* (www.motherisk.org/JFAS), a peer-reviewed journal dedicated to all aspects of FASD, offers free access to a lot of the latest studies and literature. It also contains the video-taped webcast of the 4th Annual FACE Research Roundtable, where researchers and program providers described their work in the field of FAS. The webcast also includes the TV documentary, *FAS: When the Children Grow Up*, a revealing program that tells the story of several adults living with FAS. You can view the webcast by clicking on the links at www.motherisk.org/JFAS/detail.php?id=40.

MYTHS AND FACTS ABOUT ALCOHOL AND DRUG ABUSE

Myth: Alcohol or drugs taken after the first trimester will not affect the unborn baby.

Fact: Most organ development is completed a few weeks *after* the first trimester. Brain development continues *throughout* pregnancy and after birth. Exposure to substances *any time* in the pregnancy can affect the baby's brain. Call the Motherisk Helpline at (877) 327-4636 or other teratogen center to understand the risks better.

Myth: A breastfeeding mother can provide more breast milk for her baby by drinking beer.

Fact: When a mother drinks alcohol, it passes into her breast milk. Studies have shown that infants take in less breast milk when alcohol is present. Drinking alcohol may also reduce milk flow. Call the Motherisk Helpline or other teratogen center for the facts on the effects of alcohol while breastfeeding.

Myth: Some kinds of alcohol are less harmful than others.
Fact: Any type of alcohol can harm your baby (beer, coolers, wine, or spirits). Binge drinking and heavy drinking are very harmful to an unborn baby.

Myth: One drink in pregnancy is enough to cause Fetal Alcohol Syndrome (FAS).
Fact: A safe amount of alcohol in pregnancy is not known. But a single drink before you knew you were pregnant will not cause FAS. Avoid drinking when you know you are pregnant. Call the Motherisk Helpline or other teratogen center to talk about how drinking during pregnancy can affect your unborn baby's development.

Myth: Children with FASD can grow out of their problems.
Fact: Though there are things that parents, doctors, and teachers can do to help children with FASD, it is an incurable, lifelong disorder. And as children with FASD get older, their problems can get more and more disturbing — especially once they become teenagers.

Myth: The issues of alcohol use in pregnancy and FASD are only the pregnant woman's problem.
Fact: Although a father who drinks will not cause FASD, his support and encouragement can help his partner avoid alcohol before, during her pregnancy, and while breastfeeding.

Myth: There is no hope for a baby exposed to heavy drug and alcohol use.
Fact: There is always hope. Drug and alcohol use in pregnancy affects each baby differently. Call the Motherisk Helpline or other teratogen center for information on the risks of birth defects and where to find prenatal support.

Smoking

Approximately 5.4 million people in Canada smoke. Data collected by the Canadian Tobacco Use Monitoring Survey (CTUMS) between February and December 2002 showed that approximately 23% of men and 20% of women aged 15 years and older were current smokers.

That same survey found that more than a quarter of Canadian women between the ages of 20 and 44, reported being pregnant in the last five years. Of these, 11% smoked regularly during their most recent pregnancy, and 13% reported that their spouse smoked regularly at home during that time. We suspect these percentages would be similar among pregnant women in the United States.

When you smoke, more than 1400 different chemicals enter your blood. These chemicals pass through the placenta, enter the umbilical cord, and reach your unborn child. They include carbon monoxide (the same gas that comes out of a car's exhaust pipe) and thiocyanate. These two chemicals interfere with oxygen delivery to the fetus. Smoking also delivers chemicals such as nicotine, sulfates, and lead — to mention just a few.

Some of our patients shrug off these risks. They know other women who had healthy babies in the past while smoking. But the risks to the unborn child are very real. Decreased birth weight and increased prematurity caused by smoking land many thousands of babies of smokers in neonatal intensive care and on assisted ventilation with grim consequences. Once home, the risk of Sudden Infant Death Syndrome is 1 in 1000 babies in general, but three times higher among smokers.

FACT ✔ **Help Prevent SIDS**

When you smoke, your baby smokes. Maternal smoking has been shown to decrease the body weight of the baby and to increase the risk of miscarriage, stillbirth (death of the baby after 20 weeks of pregnancy), prematurity (being born before term), and Sudden Infant Death Syndrome (SIDS). Every year in North America 1,000 babies die of SIDS because of smoking! For those who survive, long-term effects on behavior and attention span may emerge as the child becomes older.

Quitting Smoking

These hazards are potentially preventable. The best way to protect your unborn baby is to quit entirely. Cutting down is better than doing nothing. To be at all effective, a woman who is trying to reduce the number of cigarettes that she smokes or has switched to low-tar cigarettes should also be sure not to inhale more deeply or puff more often. The point is not simply to reduce the number of cigarettes, but also the amount of nicotine and other chemicals that enter your and your unborn baby's system.

Quitting before (or during pregnancy) will also prepare you for an important part of caring for your baby — breastfeeding. For most women, breastfeeding is the best way to feed a new baby. If you smoke while breastfeeding, chemicals such as nicotine can poison this important source of nourishment. The cigarette smoke itself can also harm the baby.

That said, we acknowledge that quitting smoking can be difficult. For some chronic smokers, smoking is an addiction. The body is dependent on a certain level of nicotine, and when this level falls, the body craves it. This is why so many people fail to stop smoking time after time.

Those who do quit usually have the benefit of strong motivation, effective counseling, and support. Partners, family, friends, and health-care professionals should be active participants in a process that may be hard for you, but so very important to you and your child.

SAFETY/RISK ❖ Kick the Habit

If you are a smoker, the best time to quit is when you're planning your pregnancy. If your pregnancy is unplanned, quitting within the first trimester can lower your baby's risk of low birth weight and other health complications. But it's never too late to quit. Kicking the habit, even during the late stages of pregnancy, can help your unborn baby get the oxygen needed to grow.

Smoking Cessation Programs

So where should you start? We suggest you begin with your doctor. Once you've booked that appointment with your doctor, you may also want to discuss the pros and cons of nicotine replacement therapy. Nicotine replacement therapy can come in the form of gum, spray, chewing gum or patch. The idea is to give the body the nicotine it craves, without the cigarettes. This way you receive only nicotine, at levels lower than in cigarettes, without all those other 1,400 chemicals. The dose of nicotine is decreased gradually to prevent cravings.

Nicotine replacement therapy is given free to pregnant women in France. In Canada, it is recommended by the Ontario Medical Association. In studies to-date, the nicotine patch has not been show to pose a risk in pregnancy.

RESOURCES

For more information about smoking cessation and pregnancy, visit the Pregnet website at http://pregnets.org/.

Drug Abuse

Recreational drugs have become a part of life for many women of reproductive age. While drug use is not consistent with a healthy lifestyle for the adult user, when an unborn child is involved, the risks may be much more serious.

Many women (and men) who use cocaine, amphetamines, heroin, and LSD believe they are not addicted. But if you use drugs regularly, you may be physically or psychologically dependent on them. It is important to consult a medical doctor and seek diagnosis and treatment if in fact you are drug dependent. You should also be aware that drug dependence is not limited to the use of 'street drugs' such as cocaine and ecstasy, but may also involve common medications. For example, at Motherisk we counsel large numbers of women who use Tylenol 3. They typically say that they need it for back pain and other body aches. But women and men who use Tylenol 3 continuously for weeks or months on end may in fact be feeding an addiction. Tylenol 3 contains codeine, a narcotic analgesic that is changed by the body to the highly addictive substance, morphine.

If you frequently use potentially addictive medications or recreational drugs, you may need help. Do not be embarrassed, do not postpone it for tomorrow — seek help today.

FACT ✔ **Drug Abuse Dangers**

Abuse of drugs during pregnancy may lead to premature birth, a baby who is small for gestational age, and perinatal health complications for mother and child. Drug abuse during pregnancy is also associated with higher rates of miscarriage and stillbirth (death of the fetus after 20 weeks of pregnancy). Finally, because the drugs of abuse taken by the mother reach the unborn baby, the newborn infant may suffer from a withdrawal syndrome, as the baby craves the drugs he or she was exposed to in pregnancy.

Risks

Drugs of abuse may affect the unborn baby either directly by entering into the baby's body, or indirectly, by affecting the mother's health.

In general, women who are drug dependent tend to have higher rates of health risks, especially sexually transmitted diseases, including Hepatitis B and C, HIV, gonorrhea, and syphilis. All of these diseases may transfer to the baby and endanger his or her life. Drug dependent women also tend to take less care of

---

SAFETY/RISK ❖ Get the Facts

If you have used drugs of abuse before you knew you were pregnant and have discontinued such use, and if alcohol was not part of your pattern of drug use, you have a very good chance of bearing a healthy child. However, it is important for you to seek counseling and advice from an expert. Do not let friends, family, partners, and others scare you based on what they saw on TV or what they may think. Get the facts, and nothing less.

---

their own health and seek less prenatal care during pregnancy. Drug dependent women may also be undernourished and suffer from spousal abuse and trauma. Their physical health may not be optimal.

Typically, a baby suffering from a withdrawal syndrome is irritable, cries for long hours, sweats, experiences diarrhea, and may have seizures (convulsions). The child may not be consoled by breast or formula. The treatment in most cases is to give the baby medication or the substance being craved (e.g., morphine). The amount given is tapered off gradually until the craving stops.

The most common drug of abuse consumed by women of reproductive age is tetrahydrocanabinnol, either as marijuana or hashish. Although there is no convincing evidence that such exposure increases the risks of major malformation, some recent research points to specific delays in brain development in some children.

We're learning more and more each day about the effects of specific drugs of abuse. For example, we know that cocaine raises maternal blood pressure, which in turn can cause abruption of the placenta. Abruption presents as bleeding from the placenta. This bleeding can endanger the life of the baby.

Numerous studies suggest that babies born to cocaine-using mothers have higher risk of prematurity, perinatal complications, and even more long-term effects on brain development. However, it is still not clear how much of these effects are due to the cocaine itself or to other risks, such as poverty, poor prenatal care, stress, and sexually transmitted diseases.

RESOURCES

For more information, call the Motherisk Alcohol and Substance Use Helpline to talk to a counselor at (877) 327-4636.

CHAPTER TEN

Chemical and Radiation Exposures

Q. I am a secretary in a plant that paints cars. I can often smell the turpentine and many other chemicals. I heard this could be risky to the baby.

— Motherisk Caller

A. Smelling organic solvents does not mean toxicity. The nose can smell very low concentrations in the air. With your type of exposure, it is unlikely that your unborn baby is at risk. However, most plants have regular measures of airborne levels of chemicals. You are entitled to review these numbers.

— Motherisk Counselor

Chemical Exposures At Home

Pregnant and planning women call Motherisk every day with questions about home cleaning products, paints, and other common household exposures. What we offer here are general guidelines regarding some commonly used products. We recommend, however, that you call a teratogen information counselor in your area for more detailed information.

Household Cleaning Products

Most products are safe for use as directed. Make sure, however, to use them in well-ventilated areas. Also use appropriate safeguards (such as gloves) where directed. Do not use industrial-strength products at home, and if you feel sick (e.g., dizzy or nauseous) while you're doing your cleaning, stop and consult your physician.

Interior Paints

Many pregnant women like to prepare for their child's arrival by painting one or more rooms of the house. If you decide to paint, your safest choice is latex or water-based paints. Water-based paints have low volatility and pose no increased reproductive risk. Also, be sure that the room you are painting is well ventilated. If, however, you feel sick while you're painting, stop and consult your physician. It is not recommended that you use oil-based paints.

Insecticides

Try using a mineral oil-based product such as Skin-So-Soft. If it doesn't work as effectively as you would like, choose a product that contains less than 30% DEET, and use it sparingly. You'll have to read the product label carefully.

Pesticides

It is probably best to avoid these products, if possible. If the interior of your home must be sprayed, stay out of the home two to three times longer than recommended by the pesticide manufacturer. Have someone open the windows after spraying, in order to ventilate the area well. If a pesticide is applied to your lawn, do not walk on the grass for the recommended amount of time.

Poisoning in Pregnancy

Throughout this book we have considered what happens to the fetus and mother when medications are in used in appropriate and prescribed doses. However, there are cases in which women may be poisoned by an overdose. In fact, such cases are not rare.

First Aid

The first principle is to rescue the mother by either preventing the absorption of the medicine or chemical into her body, or facilitating its exit from the body. For selected drugs, there are antidotes, that is, specific medications that neutralize their action in different ways. Call your local poison control center for up-to-date information on symptoms and antidotes.

A second important principle is to monitor closely the well-being of the fetus. Large studies show that in most cases, when the mother is rescued, the baby will be all right.

Carbon Monoxide

There are, however, cases where the fetus is in danger even when the mother is not. For example, carbon monoxide poisoning can occur where there is incomplete combustion of fuel in furnaces, on boats, and elsewhere.

Every winter scores of people are poisoned by carbon monoxide, and some of them may be pregnant women. Carbon monoxide sticks to hemoglobin in the blood, inhibiting its ability to carry oxygen. The affect on the fetus is aggravated by the fact that certain differences in fetal hemoglobin allow carbon monoxide to persist at higher levels and for a longer period of time than in adult hemoglobin. The result is that the fetus may sustain damage even if the mother recovers totally from the poisoning.

Cosmetic Hair Treatments

I usually have my color done every couple of months, but now that I'm pregnant I'm worried about how it may affect my baby. What do you know about hair dyes in pregnancy?

Hair treatments involve many different chemicals and degrees of exposure. What's more, manufacturers often change formulations, making it very hard to know exactly what your exposure during pregnancy may be. As a result, there's not a lot of available safety data regarding their use in pregnancy. While your best bet is to call your local teratogen information service on a product-by-product basis, we can answer some basic questions here.

In-Depth

What we know about the risk or safety of permanent hair dyes comes from two sources: animal studies and reports from women who dyed their hair during pregnancy. In animal studies, pregnant animal subjects were exposed to doses 100 times higher than would normally be used on humans, and no significant changes were seen in the fetus's development.

Meanwhile, though we know that many women who are pregnant choose to dye their hair, there are no known reports of harm to the fetus. We also know that only a small amount of the dye applied to the scalp is absorbed into the system (and later excreted into the urine). Very little is available to the fetus.

Permanents

Again, the safety data on 'perms' available to us is derived from animal studies. The waving solution (an alkaline thioglycolate solution) may irritate the skin, and the fixation solution (an acid hydrogen peroxide solution) may cause respiratory symptoms, but these have not been associated with other effects and very little of the product is absorbed into the system. Occasional use in a well-ventilated area is *probably safe.*

SAFETY/RISK ❖ Be Extra Safe

Putting all the research pieces together (animal study data, plus lack of known reports from exposed pregnant women, plus data regarding minimal absorption through the skin), it would appear that occasional use of permanent hair dyes in a well-ventilated area is unlikely to be a concern during pregnancy. If, however, you want to be extra safe, you may want to choose a hair coloring process, such as highlights, where the chemicals don't touch the scalp.

Straightening

Here, we actually have a study in humans that addressed two specific questions regarding the effects of straighteners during pregnancy. In this study, the use of straightening products was not found to increase the chance of low birth weight or preterm delivery. However, the study did not look at the risk of other potential hazards, such as birth defects. Nonetheless, the reasoning applied to the use of permanent hair dyes during pregnancy will apply to hair straighteners. Only a small amount of hair straightening product is actually absorbed into the system. That means that the developing fetus will only be exposed to a very small amount. Occasional use in a well-ventilated area is *probably safe.*

Bleaching

Hair bleaching formulas contain hydrogen peroxide and 'per-' salt, such as ammonium persulfate. In most cases, the level of exposure is very low. However, some people are hypersensitive to these agents and may experience contact allergy, rhinitis, or respiratory symptoms. If you experience such a reaction, you should see your physician. There are no reports of reproductive effects in either humans or animals.

Chemical Exposures At Work

Today, more and more women are working in industries where they may be exposed to chemicals in the workplace. You may be one of them. With exposure come concerns about fetal safety when the exposure occurs during pregnancy.

FACT ✔ **Chemicals Not Tested**

There are thousands of industrial chemicals in use. Unlike medicinal drugs that have to be tested in pregnant animals before being placed on the market, no such tests are required for chemicals. As a result, you may be working with chemicals that have not been tested to determine their fetal safety. Without such testing, you may not be able to find the definitive answer to the question, Is it safe for my baby?

Chemical exposures that may not affect immediate maternal health may have serious consequences for the fetus. Two important examples are lead and organic solvents. Lead levels of 10 micrograms per deciliter are not likely to harm you; they can, however, affect the IQ of the unborn baby. Similarly, airborne levels of organic solvents that may not affect your health may affect the development of the baby's vision. So, it is important to learn more about the known risks of certain chemical exposures in your workplace.

If you are working with or around chemicals, it is very likely that your employer maintains data safety sheets that describe the limit of safe adult exposure. You should ask to see and read these data safety sheets.

It is also likely that the air levels of chemicals are measured and recorded periodically. During pregnancy (as well as before or after pregnancy) you are entitled to know the levels of exposures that have been measured in your workplace. Once you've gathered as much information and data as possible, speak to your employer's occupational health director or nurse. You may also want to consult a Motherisk counselor or other teratogen information specialist in your area.

SAFETY/RISK ◆ **Potential Harm**

Sometimes the proper use of masks, ventilating hoods, and other protective devices may be enough to protect you and your baby from potential harm. If not, you and your employer may want to consider a move to another area or department for the duration of your pregnancy. But be sure to consider all the available facts before deciding to continue or quit working.

CHEMICAL SAFETY/RISK DEFINITIONS

The United States Occupational Safety and Health Administrations and the Ministry of Labour in Canada have adopted the same recommendations in setting and enforcing workplace standards. The administration receives guidance from the National Institute for Occupational Safety and Health and the American Conference of Government Industrial Hygienists. These organizations do not differentiate between pregnant and non-pregnant women in their recommendations.

As a rule, available safety information is about the health of adults working with the particular chemical, not the health of the fetus. Because the fetus is rapidly developing, it may be sensitive to low levels of exposure that are not likely to affect your own health.

Here are some definitions of exposures, as they are used by different professional organizations and regulatory agencies.

Airborne Levels

PEL: "Permissible Exposure Limits" as set by the U.S. Occupational Safety and Health Administration (OSHA).

TLV: "Threshold Limit Value" as set by the American Conference of Governmental Industrial Hygienists (ACGIH). Threshold limit values (TLV) can refer to a time-weighted average (TWA), a short-term exposure limit (STEL), or a ceiling (C).

REL: "Recommended Exposure Limit" as set by the U.S. National Institute for Occupational Safety and Health (NIOH).

STEL: "Short Term Exposure Limit."

All four (PEL, TLV, REL, STEL) relate to airborne levels (levels in the air) that a worker can be exposed to at work, day after a day, without risking potential health problems. These limits and values represent "safe" levels. But remember that the safety was measured in adults, not in unborn babies.

Time-Weighted Averages

TWA: "Time-weighted average" levels of a chemical for a normal 8-hour workday or a 40-hour work week which is not toxic to most workers.

Units

When talking about exposure in air, the unit of measurement is typically parts per million (ppm) or parts per billion.

Risk

TLV-TWA is an average concentration for a normal 8-hour day and 40-hour week to which workers can be exposed without adverse effect.

TLV-STEL is the maximum concentration acceptable during a 15-minute period during an 8-hour day. It should occur no more than four times daily with an hour between exposures.

TLV-C is the maximum allowable airborne concentration at any time during an 8-hour work period; it should not be exceeded.

IDLH is "immediately dangerous to life and health."

Guide to Safety/Risk of Common Occupational Chemicals

The following list summarizes what is currently known about the safety of selected occupational chemicals in humans. Each statement includes the workplace standard for healthy *adults*, and tells you the maximum exposure that will not adversely affect your health. Unfortunately, there are no similar standards for the pregnant woman that accurately reflect exposures that are safe for the fetus.

CHEMICAL	WHAT IS CURRENTLY KNOWN
Anesthetic Gases TLV: 50 ppm REL-TWA: 25 ppm	Gases used in surgery to induce sleep during operations are, of course, an occupational exposure for female anesthetists, doctors, and other female operating room staff. In fact, the majority of staff in operating rooms are women. All of the common gases, including nitrous oxide, enflurence, and halothane, do not cause malformations during a single exposure (i.e., one operation). However, repeated studies suggest that they increase the risk of miscarriage among women exposed occupationally. During pregnancy, it is recommended that operating room staff try to minimize such exposure.
Carbon Monoxide TLV-TWA: 25 ppm	Carbon monoxide is produced from the incomplete combustion of fuels. Acute poisoning can result from faulty furnaces and engines and can lead to loss of consciousness and death due to the binding of carbon monoxide to hemoglobin, inhibiting the transfer of oxygen to the body. Chronic mild exposure occurs with cigarette smoking and may occur in industry. One such example involves methylene chloride, which is broken down to carbon monoxide. The possibility of increased risk of miscarriages has been discussed, as well as reduced sperm concentrations. Acute poisoning may cause brain damage.

CHEMICAL	WHAT IS CURRENTLY KNOWN
Cholinesterase Inhibitors TLV-TWA: 0.1 mg/m^2 for parathion	These appear mostly as pesticides (e.g., malathion, parathion, diazinon). In animals, exposure to high doses damages the fetus. Women working in production of organophosphates or in agriculture should monitor their levels of erythrocyte and plasma cholinesterase.
Epichlorhydrin TLV-TWA: 0.5 ppm	This compound is a suspected mutagen (causing gene mutations) and carcinogen (inducing cancer). In animals, it has been shown to damage the testicle of the adult male who works with the compound.
Ethylene Dibromide (Dibromoethane) PEL-TWA: 20 ppm	Decreased sperm counts were noticed in some studies of men exposed to this chemical in agricultural work.
Ethylene Oxide TLV-TWA: 1 ppm	Ethylene oxide is a suspected carcinogen (inducing cancer). One study found more miscarriages among hospital workers exposed to 0.1 to 0.5 ppm over an 8-hour work day, on a regular basis.
Formaldehyde TLV: 0.3 ppm PEL-TWA: 1 ppm	Increased miscarriages were described among cosmetologists and laboratory workers.
Halogenated Hydrocarbons Solvents – Chloroprene TLV-TWA: 10 ppm	Impotence and decreased libido were described in men.
Lead TLV-TWA: 0.5 mg/m^2	May increase miscarriage rate and prematurity. May affect fetal brain development when maternal blood levels are above 10 mg/dL.
Mercury TLV-TWA: 0.01 mg/m^3	Organic mercury and mostly methyl and ethyl mercury have been shown to accumulate in the fetal brain and cause various degrees of brain damage in newborns and children.
Organic Solvents	This wide group of compounds is used to dissolve organic materials in many industries. They include such well-known compounds as toluene and benzene, as well as hundreds of other chemicals. They have been shown to increase the risk of malformations in general, and the risk of brain function in particular. Workplace levels that cause pregnant women to have such symptoms as burning eyes, cough, or breathing difficulties are associated with higher fetal risks.
Organochlorine Insecticides	Chemicals such as lindane may cause menstrual problems and infertility.
Polychlorinated Biphenyls (PCBs)	One study found that poisoning (through contaminated rice) caused stillbirth, neonatal skin problems, low birth weight, and developmental problems. However, these findings are most probably not valid for low-level environmental exposure.

Occupational Exposure to Mercury

Q *I'm a dental hygienist and I use mercury in the dentist's office where I work. My partner and I have decided we would like to have a child and so I'm planning to get pregnant. I'm doing lots of reading and understand that mercury could affect my baby. I have no symptoms of mercury toxicity. What should I do?*

A Ask your family physician to arrange for you to be tested for levels of mercury in whole blood and, preferably, in urine. These tests will confirm your actual exposure. If you have significant exposure, you'll want to put off getting pregnant until your body has eliminated it from your system. It will also be important to know what the airborne concentration of mercury is in your workplace. Currently, mercury vapor concentrations greater than 0.01 mg/m^3 are considered unsafe. Also, women of childbearing age should avoid contact with mercury salts in the workplace.

In-Depth

Mercury toxicity has been recognized for centuries; it is referred to in the works of Hippocrates. The first indication of fetal toxicity occurred when women undergoing mercury treatment for syphilis were noted to have frequent abortions. Our current understanding about the effects of the mercury during pregnancy is based on reports of human mercury poisoning during pregnancy, and what we know about the sources of mercury exposure, how pregnant women absorb mercury, the ability of mercury compounds to pass through the placenta, and the amount that is likely to enter the fetus's blood and circulation systems.

Clinical Reports of Human Fetal Poisoning

In 1953, in Minamata, Japan, neurologic manifestations, including mental confusion, convulsions, and coma, were reported in villagers who had eaten methylmercury-contaminated fish and shellfish (38% of them later died). Between 1953 and 1971, cerebral palsy, chorea, ataxia, tremors, seizures, and mental retardation were seen in the children of exposed mothers. The infants had not eaten contaminated fish, so the neurologic symptoms must have resulted from toxicity *in utero*.

In 1964, an epidemic similar to the one in Minamata occurred in Niigata, Japan. The source of methylmercury was traced to ingestion of fish contaminated by mercury from industrial discharge.

In 1968, 10 cases of prenatal poisoning in mothers who ingested grain treated with methylmercury were reported from the Soviet Union. Severe mental retardation was described in three cases and decreased birth weight and muscle tone were noted in others. Isolated cases have been reported from Lund, Sweden; King County, Washington; and Alamogordo, New Mexico.

In 1971, a widespread epidemic with similar symptoms occurred in Iraq. The source was barley and wheat grain treated with methylmercury for defumigation and distributed in error among Iraqi farmers.

Types and Sources of Exposure

There are various types of mercury: metallic mercury, mercury salts, and organic mercurials (methylmercury and phenylmercury).

Contamination of inland and coastal waterways is usually caused by pollution from natural and industrial sources. Microorganisms in river and lake sediments convert various inorganic and organic mercurials into the most toxic mercury compound, methylmercury, which is taken in by fish. Methylmercury in fish accumulates to concentrations thousands of times greater than in the surrounding water.

FACT ✔ Dietary Intake

Dietary intake is the most important source of environmental exposure to mercury, with fish and other seafood products being the main sources of mercury in the diet. Environmental exposure can also occur at home (rooms painted with latex paints that contain mercury pigments or fungicides), in areas of industrial pollution, and in agricultural work through seed treatment. Occupational exposure is higher in certain professions, such as dentistry, paint production, and the amalgamations industry. The source of mercury for most of the general population and for those exposed at work (including dentists and dental staff) is metallic (inorganic) mercury.

Maternal Absorption and Distribution

Mercury is absorbed through the lungs, gastrointestinal (GI) tract, and skin. Though mercury can be absorbed through the skin, this process is too slow to be of much importance, especially for acute exposures. Mercuric ions ($Hg2+$) are more readily absorbed through the GI tract.

Organic mercury is absorbed to an even greater extent than inorganic salts. Most (80% to 100%) of these compounds are absorbed by the GI tract, but much is subsequently secreted in the bile. The vapor of organic mercurials readily diffuses through lung alveoli. The skin can also absorb these compounds, particularly through sores or wounds.

Metallic mercury (HgO) diffuses more readily across cell membranes. It is distributed more widely than the ionic form and can penetrate into the brain, attaining concentrations 10 times those of mercuric compounds.

Placental Transfer

Mercury compounds can pass through the placenta into the blood of the fetus. The effect on the fetus depends on how readily these compounds penetrate the placental membranes and how much they accumulate within the fetus's central nervous system.

For metallic mercury, up to 0.22% of the mercury vapor inhaled by mother rats was present in fetal tissues 24 hours after exposure. It is apparent that, while placental cells can readily accumulate mercuric ions, relatively small amounts of these compounds enter the fetus's blood. Methylmercury, the more toxic form, passes more readily through placental tissues and enters the fetus's circulation systems.

Symptoms

Acute inhalation of high concentrations of metallic mercury vapor leads to severe inflammation of the lung and pulmonary edema. Chronic intoxication from inhaling mercury vapor results in tremor, neuropsychiatric disturbances (fatigue, insomnia, anorexia, memory loss), and gingivostomatitis (inflammation of gum tissue).

Diagnosis

Whole blood and, preferably, urine tests for levels of mercury are useful for confirming exposure. Urine and blood tests can be ordered by family physicians; tests are done at public health laboratories.

Preventive Measures

Prevention, the best management strategy in occupational settings, can be done through environmental monitoring and decontamination procedures, such as:

- having appropriate ventilation in work areas to prevent toxic accumulation;
- routinely sampling personal and area air in the environment;
- monitoring mercury levels through industrial hygiene surveys;
- testing for ambient air concentrations, which can be detected at levels as low as 0.001 mg/m^3; and
- carrying out mercury decontamination procedures in buildings by removing carpets; cleaning floors, walls, and solid surfaces several times with a product containing a metallic mercury sulfide-converting powder, a chelating compound, and a dispersing agent; and applying a polyurethane coating to all floor surfaces.

RECOMMENDED MERCURY TLV-TWA VALUES

Recommended TLV-TWA for mercury vapor and for inorganic and non-alkaline organic mercurials are shown in this table

An air concentration of 0.05 mgHg/m^3 after long-term exposure corresponds to a urine concentration of 50 µg/L (normal value less than 10 to 20 µg/L) and blood concentration of 30 to 35 µg/L (normal value less than 20 µg/L). The Environmental Protection Agencies suggested ambient air level for population exposure is less than 1 µgHg/m^3. In Russia, TLV-C values are much lower than those recommended in North America: 0.01 mgHg/m^3 for mercury vapor ($^1/_{10}$ of the U.S. recommendations) and 0.005 mgHg/m^3 for alkyl mercury ($^1/_8$ th of the U.S. recommendations).

Note: µg = microgram m = meter.

Values	Mercury Vapor / Inorganic and Non-Alkaline Organic Mercurials	Ethyl and Methyl Mercury
Threshold Limit Value (time-weighted average)	0.05 µg/m^3	0.01 µg/m^3
Threshold Limit Value (ceiling)	0.1 µg/m^3	0.04 µg/m^3
Short-Term Exposure Limit	0.03 µg/m^3	0.03 µg/m^3
Immediately Dangerous to Life and Health	No data	10 µg/m^3

Radiation and Electromagnetic Exposures

Diagnostic Radiation

X-ray examination is often required to diagnose a variety of medical conditions. This can be a dental x-ray, a chest radiograph, or computed tomography (CT or CAT) scan. A radionuclide isotope may also be required to scan the thyroid, bones, or other organs.

Our knowledge about the effects of radiation in pregnancy is based, in part, on lessons learned during World War II. Thousands of people were exposed to radiation when the atomic bomb was dropped on Hiroshima and Nagasaki. Some of the exposed were pregnant women. These tragic events led to a better understanding of the fetal effects of radiation and how much exposure results in fetal damage.

Units of radiation are expressed in 'rads.' It appears that the adverse effects on the fetus (mostly on brain development) became apparent when the fetus was exposed to 20 rads or more. Just to be on the safe side, we now use 5 rads as the 'safety limit' in pregnancy.

SAFETY/RISK ❖ Conservative Approach

Almost all diagnostic procedures result in fetal exposure that is substantially lower than 5 rads. Still, we believe that a conservative approach to diagnostic radiation in pregnancy is best. If you plan to have an x-ray, it is important to ensure (by pregnancy test) that you have not conceived.If you have conceived, the x-ray should not be aimed at the abdomen, and it is important to use a lead apron to prevent most of the radiation from reaching the uterus. If you are exposed to diagnostic radiation in pregnancy and wish to determine the amount of possible exposure to the fetus, the radiologist who did the test should tell you the estimated amount of radiation emitted.

Radioisotopes

Exposure to radioisotopes (radioactive tracers) is more complicated because there are scores of different ones. Again, in general the amount of radiation emitted at the fetus is small. Nonetheless, there is a concern that these compounds may concentrate in the fetal tissue and eventually cause damage.

A common example is radioactive iodine, which may be given to the mother to diagnose or treat a thyroid condition.

ESTIMATED FETAL RADIATION DOSES DURING DIAGNOSTIC X-RAYS

This table shows how many rads the fetus is exposed to in selected examples of diagnostic x-ray procedures. Note: 1,000 millirads = 1 rad. up to 5 rads is considered safe in pregnancy.

Examination Procedure	Estimated Fetal Dose (millirads)
X-ray	
Upper Gastrointestinal Series	100 millirads
Cholecystography	100 millirads
Lumbar Spine Radiography	400 millirads
Pelvic Radiography	200 millirads
Hip and Femur Radiography	300 millirads
Retrograde Pyelography	600 millirads
Abdominal (kidneys, uterus, bladder) Radiography	250 millirads
Lumbar Spine: Anteroposterior	750 millirads
Lumbar Spine: Lateral	91 millirads
Lumbar Spine: Oblique	100 millirads
Computed Tomography (CAT Scan)	
Head	0
Chest	16 millirads
Abdomen	3,000 millirads

The radioactive iodine crosses the placenta and may concentrate in the thyroid gland of the fetus, potentially damaging it. The good news is that the thyroid in a fetus begins to be functional only after 2 months of pregnancy. Therefore, an earlier exposure (say, at 4 weeks) will not remain long enough to concentrate in the fetal thyroid gland.

Again, if you plan to receive radioactive isotopes, it is best to rule out pregnancy. If you are exposed to radioisotopes in pregnancy, it is important to know which kind of compound you received and at what dose. The experts will be able to calculate the potential exposure to the fetus.

Exposure to Electromagnetic Fields

Q I heard on the radio that working with home appliances could increase the risk of miscarriages. What is your advice?

A Two studies from California suggested an increased risk of miscarriages associated with exposure to magnetic fields. Even if the threshold associated with such risk is a true risk (and not just an *association*), it does not appear to arise from typical use of hair dryers, microwave ovens, vacuum cleaners, and similar home appliances.

In-Depth

We are all surrounded by the magnetic fields of scores of appliances and other electric devices we use routinely. Currently, there is no strong biologic indication or study result to suggest that electromagnetic fields encountered in day-to-day life affect our reproductive systems adversely. During the 1980s, when video display terminals became part of life, there were high levels of anxiety among pregnant women, some of whom were told to wear lead aprons at work 8 hours a day for 9 months. This issue was put to rest by the low levels of electromagnetism shown to be emitted by video display terminals and the negative results of epidemiologic studies.

Studies of Exposure

Several studies have reported varying results concerning the association between exposure to the electromagnetic fields of home and personal use appliances and rates of miscarriage. For example, in 2000, a group of researchers showed that users of electric bed heaters did not have more spontaneous abortions than those who did not use them. This was true for both electric blankets and waterbeds.

Another study showed an association between peak-per-day levels above 16 milligaus (gaus is the unit used to measure electromagnetic energy) and miscarriage. Cumulative exposure did not yield a similar association. However, study design and potential confounders (other plausible explanations for the observed outcomes) undercut the strength of these findings. For a fuller discussion of this and other studies, read the

> **SAFETY/RISK**
>
> **Reassurance**
> When we interpret the evidence, we understand that it is reasonable to expect more and better controlled data, but in the meantime, we can reassure you that it is safe to continue regular use of home appliances.

February 2003 Motherisk Update, posted on the Motherisk website (www.motherisk.org) in the 'Update' archives.

So, what can we tell pregnant women who are afraid to dry their hair or make toast for their children? Let us assume a worst-case scenario (i.e., that the data are biologically true, and that a peak level of 16 mG is the threshold for risk for expectant women). Now, consider the following. The amount of exposure depends on how far the body is from the source. When used normally, hair dryers aimed at the head are at least 60 cm from the uterus. At this distance, peak uterine exposure to an electromagnetic field is so small it cannot be detected. Microwave ovens are typically at least 70 to 80 cm from the body of someone pushing the buttons. At that distance, the electromagnetic dose to the skin is less than 10 mG, and the dose that will reach the uterus is much lower. Vacuum cleaners are typically at least 60 cm from a user's abdomen, and the dose is similar for typical use: less than 10 mG and probably much lower.

Electric Shock

Q *When I was 23 weeks pregnant, I experienced a minor electric shock while using my hair dryer. I felt the current in my right hand. I was wearing shoes. I went to the emergency room of our local hospital, was observed there for several hours, and then discharged home. Is my fetus at risk now or later in the pregnancy?*

A There are conflicting reports on how harmful electric shock is to a fetus. Several factors, such as the magnitude of the current and the duration of contact, are thought to affect outcome. In this case, it appears the current did not travel through your abdomen. Pregnant women suffering electric shock from low-voltage current, especially the 110-V current used in North America, which did not pass through the uterus and had no or minor adverse effects on the mother, would likely have no immediate effect on a fetus. Nonetheless, fetal monitoring may be recommended.

In-Depth

Injuries from electric shock account for about 1,000 deaths annually in the United States and about 5% of admissions to burn centers. Electrocution is the fifth leading cause of fatal occupational injuries in the United States; 1% of household accidental deaths are caused by electrical injuries. More than 60% of reported electrical injuries are due to electrocution with 110- or 220-V current and most commonly result from failure to ground tools or appliances properly or from using electrical devices near water.

Injuries from accidental electrical shock range from a transient unpleasant sensation after exposure to low-intensity current to sudden death due to cardiac arrest. The effects are sometimes seen immediately after contact, but might not become apparent until several hours after injury.

Several case reports and small case series of serious complications, including fetal death, following electric shock have been published. But since reports of adverse outcomes are more often published than reports of normal outcomes, the literature does not reflect the usual outcome of contact with low-voltage current.

One researcher reviewed the cases of four women who experienced electric shock during pregnancy. All four fetuses died: one due to spontaneous abortion in the first trimester; two ceased moving immediately after the injury and were aborted; and one died 3 days after delivery with burn marks on his body. Another researcher reviewed a series of studies of 15 victims of electric shock during pregnancy published in the English literature. The fetuses died in 73% of cases, and there was only one normal pregnancy outcome. Yet another group of researchers reported on six pregnant women who suffered electric shock at home. In all cases, the current went from the hand to the foot, probably through the uterus, and all of the women felt fine after the incident. Three fetuses were stillborn, two within a week of the electric shock and one after 12 weeks. All had severe intrauterine growth retardation.

Motherisk published one prospective cohort study of pregnant women who experienced electric shock. Our results somewhat contradict previous findings. Of 31 pregnant women who called us, 28 were exposed to electric shock while using home appliances. Twenty-eight of these women delivered healthy newborns. One baby had a ventricular septal defect (a common congenital heart defect) that closed spontaneously during early childhood, and two women had spontaneous abortions, one temporally related to the accidental injury, the other probably not associated with it. We found no differences in mean birth weight, gestational age at delivery, rates of cesarean section, or neonatal distress between electric-shock and control groups.

Risk Factors

The pathway along which the current traveled probably has the greatest effect on the outcome of pregnancy. The passage of current from hand to foot through the uterus could cause sudden contraction of the uterus. Amniotic fluid transmits current effectively, and this could increase risk of spontaneous abortions and fetal burns or death. Another confirmation of this is the relatively benign effects on fetuses of the electroconvulsive therapy (ECT) used to treat depression and psychosis during all three trimesters of pregnancy. During ECT, the current does not travel through the uterus.

Possible blunt trauma to the uterus after loss of consciousness and a fall is also of concern and illustrates the need to monitor both mother and fetus.

Duration of current flow in the body, body weight, and being wet during the electrical injury are also risk factors for more severe adverse outcomes.

Surveillance

Although fetal and obstetric surveillance are recommended following electrical injury, there is no evidence that any form of monitoring or treatment has a direct effect on outcome.

Recommendations for fetal monitoring after electric shock have been published. Before 20 weeks gestation, no monitoring is needed. During the second half of pregnancy, fetal echocardiography is recommended if not performed earlier, and maternal electrocardiography (ECG) and fetal heart rate and uterine activity monitoring are recommended for 24 hours if the injury involved loss of consciousness, abnormal maternal ECG results, or known maternal cardiovascular illness. Any mechanical injury to the mother (i.e., a fall) is an indication for 4 hours of fetal and uterine monitoring.

> **SAFETY/RISK**
>
> **Still Controversial**
> Pregnant women suffering electric shock from low-voltage current, especially the 110-V current used in North America, which did not pass through the uterus and had no or minor adverse effects on the mother, would likely have no immediate effect on a fetus. Nonetheless, the effect of electrical injury on the outcome of pregnancy is still controversial, and only larger prospective observational studies could give us a better understanding of expected outcomes and requirements for monitoring.

RESOURCES

Workplace Reproductive Health, Research and Strategies. Best Start: Ontario's Maternal Newborn and Early Child Development Resource Centre, 2001.

CHAPTER ELEVEN

Medical Conditions and Infections

Q. *We have had a cat for 8 years. Honey is part of our family. But my mother-in-law says cats are dangerous during pregnancy because of this nasty infection. The idea of giving away Honey is heartbreaking. Is there any other solution?*

— Motherisk Caller

A. *Your mother-in-law means that cats may carry toxoplasmosis. If this microbe infects a pregnant woman, it can damage the baby. Since toxoplasmosis is in the cat stool, the logical solution is to avoid any contact with the cat's litter box. There is no need to get rid of Honey.*

— Motherisk Counselor

Women of reproductive age may suffer from chronic conditions that started long before pregnancy. For example, women with allergies or rheumatoid arthritis may have been taking medications for months or years before getting pregnant. Even without pre-existing conditions, pregnancy may cause you to suffer from conditions such as morning sickness, urinary tract infection, or gestational diabetes.

Risk Assessment

Chapter 6 of this book discusses the safety or risk of medications that you may need for pre-existing conditions or those that may arise during pregnancy. However, it is also important to talk to your doctor about the potential risks associated with the medical conditions themselves, since the risks of some untreated conditions in pregnancy may be higher than the potential risks of the medications used to control them.

Unreasonable Risk

For example, if you have asthma, it is important that your condition is well controlled during pregnancy. Uncontrolled asthma is associated with a higher risk for prematurity and other pregnancy complications, such as stillbirth. Asthma attacks during pregnancy can also deprive oxygen to the fetus and compromise the health of your baby. Most first-line asthma drugs, including betamimetic drugs (e.g., Ventolin) and inhaled steroids (e.g., Beclomethasone) have not been shown to cause major malformations in humans. That means that a pregnant woman who decides not to treat her asthma may be taking an unreasonable risk. The better course is to consult your doctor to determine which medications are best for you during pregnancy and lactation.

Another very important example is clinical depression. Depression in pregnancy is associated with higher obstetrical complications and preterm deliveries. A review of 11 studies has also shown that depressed women have 45% more miscarriages. They are also more likely to smoke, drink, and not seek prenatal care. What's more, depression in pregnancy is a strong predictor of postpartum depression.

Abrupt Discontinuation

Discontinuing medications abruptly is also a concern. In 2001, Motherisk published a study documenting the adverse effects of 36 women who called the Motherisk Program after abruptly discontinuing either antidepressants or benzodiazepines (28 had discontinued the medications on the advice of their physicians). Before becoming pregnant, these women had been functioning well with their depression controlled. They stopped the medication only because they feared it would harm their babies.

All the women suffered abrupt discontinuation syndrome; 11 subsequently reported suicidal thoughts; and four were later hospitalized. One of the remaining women had a therapeutic abortion, and one substituted alcohol for a benzodiazepine. After counseling, two-thirds restarted their medication within several days. There were no birth defects among any of the babies born to those mothers who restarted their medication.

SAFETY/RISK

Discontinuing Medications

What you need is expert advice based on your specific medical condition and history, so be sure to consult your physician or other health-care provider before discontinuing any medication you are taking. They should be able to advise you which medication is best for the control of your condition in pregnancy.

Exposure to Chicken Pox

Q I'm a kindergarten teacher and about to start a new school year. I am pregnant and expected to deliver sometime in the spring. I have heard that exposure to chicken pox can be very dangerous. What should I do if I come in contact with a child (or children) in my classroom who later come down with chickenpox?

A First, find out whether you are immune. Whether or not you had chickenpox in childhood often does not accurately determine your immunity. A rapid test, such as the latex agglutination test (LA), is useful. If test results are negative, or if testing is not feasible, varicella zoster immunoglobulin (VZIG) should be administered within 96 hours of exposure.

In-Depth

Exposure to chicken pox (varicella) is a frequent concern among pregnant women. In one 10-month period, Motherisk received 770 calls about chicken pox.

In North America most women are immune to varicella; most had chicken pox during childhood even if they do not remember having it. A study by Motherisk showed that 70% of those with a 'negative history' were in fact immune. Women of other origins have lower rates of immunity (e.g., in the West Indies it is 50%).

Adults are at higher risk of complications due to chicken pox than children are, so it is recommended that all pregnant women whose immune status is not known receive VZIG, a blood product containing antibodies against chicken pox, within 96 hours of exposure. Researchers think that VZIG helps prevent or modify the course of mothers' chicken pox infection without harming their fetuses. In an observational study, no cases of congenital varicella embryopathy were detected in 97 pregnant women who received VZIG, while 30 were found among 1500 women who did not receive VZIG.

FACT ✔ **Congenital Varicella Syndrome**

Exposure during the first 20 weeks of pregnancy can result in congenital varicella syndrome in an estimated 2% to 3% of fetuses. The syndrome is characterized by serious limb malformations, skin scarring, neurologic abnormalities (microcephaly, mental retardation, cortical atrophy, dysfunction of bowel or bladder sphincters), and eye defects.

Fifth Disease (Erythema infectiosum)

Q I'm currently 14 weeks pregnant. I'm a teacher in Grade 1, and there is an epidemic of Fifth Disease in the school where I teach. Can this disease affect my pregnancy, and if so, how should I protect myself?

A Erythema infectiosum (Fifth Disease) is usually a benign disease for children and mothers, but might have serious consequences for a fetus due to hemolytic anemia, although the risk is very low. You should evaluate your immune status. If you are already immune (IgG positive), the risks are nil. If you are not immune (although the risk of the fetus being affected is very low), fetal surveillance by repeated ultrasonographic examination and immune status re-evaluation has been recommended. If a fetus is found to be affected, intrauterine evaluation and treatment are available at tertiary care centers.

In-Depth

Human Parvovirus B19 infection occurs worldwide, most commonly among children 5 to 14 years old. The most common manifestation in children is erythema infectiosum (Fifth Disease), which typically attacks in the winter and spring. It usually involves the respiratory system, but vertical transmission (mother to fetus) occurs during pregnancy. When vertical transmission occurs during the first 20 weeks of pregnancy, the risk of developing fetal hydrops (swelling) is about 10%; the rate decreases during the second half of pregnancy.

The virus is present in the bloodstream about 7 days after inoculation and persists for 4 days. The rash typically appears 16 days after inoculation or 5 days after the virus disappears from the blood. Presence of immunoglobulin G (IgG) and absence of immune globulin M (IgM) in the blood confirms immunity. Up to 50% of adults acquire immunity during childhood, so 50% of women remain susceptible to Parvovirus B19 infection during pregnancy. The organism is highly infectious, and up to 50% of susceptible household contacts will become infected when exposed to this childhood disease. Schoolteachers who show a negative reaction to a test on blood serum and are exposed during an epidemic have a 20% to 30% chance of developing the disease.

FACT ✔ **Fifth Disease Symptoms**

Diagnosis of Fifth Disease (Erythema infectiosum) in children is generally made based on the highly characteristic 'slapped-cheeks' facial rash. The rash usually begins on the cheeks and then spreads to the trunk and limbs. Adults usually do not have a rash; the disease manifests with fever, arthralgia, adenopathy, and mild arthritis, particularly in the wrists, interphalangeal joints, and knees.

Up to 20% of the population has evidence of seroconversion (development of detectable antibodies in the blood directed against the infection) without any clinical manifestations. Some patients have only a mild respiratory illness and no rash. Children with Fifth Disease are unlikely to be infectious after the rash appears.

The infection sometimes affects other cell lines, including the white cell line and the platelets. Mild anemia is found in healthy older children and adults, but anemia can be severe in neonates. Other organs, such as the heart, liver, and spleen, can also be affected.

Effects on the Pregnancy and the Fetus

Despite earlier reports of high rates of vertical transmission, illness, and death, more recent reports demonstrate that, in most cases, no adverse effects on the fetus are evident. The vertical transmission rate is reported as 16% when mothers are infected during the first 20 weeks of gestation and 35% when mothers are infected after 20 weeks of gestation. In a prospective study, 1610 women were enrolled, and 60 (3.7%) developed detectable antibodies during pregnancy. Only 30% of these 60 women reported signs or symptoms of the disease; five had spontaneous miscarriages, but evidence of the virus was found in the fetal tissue of only one of the fetuses. The remaining 55 infected women delivered 56 healthy infants.

FACT ✔ **In Most Cases**

Research indicates that while Parvovirus infection during pregnancy can cause miscarriage and fetal hydrops that can deteriorate to fetal death, in most cases no adverse fetal effects occur.

Diagnostic Tests

Pregnant women who are not immune to the infection should reduce their exposure to sick children, especially if they are schoolteachers or daycare staff, and more so during a Fifth Disease epidemic. If they have already been exposed and the child's diagnosis has been confirmed, they should be evaluated for immune status. Neither antiviral medications nor a vaccine are available yet.

Surveillance and Treatment

Unlike some other infections during pregnancy (toxoplasmosis, syphilis, rubella, cytomegalovirus), Parvovirus is not associated with congenital malformations. Follow-up should continue for 12 weeks after diagnosis of maternal infection with biweekly ultrasound and fetal heart rate monitoring.

For fetal hydrops and with evidence of fetal anemia, fetal blood transfusion should be performed. If an affected fetus is older than 34 weeks gestation, delivery should be considered, although recently, late third-trimester intrauterine transfusions have been advocated to provide fetuses with optimal hematologic conditions before delivery. If there is evidence of intrauterine recovery, it is reasonable to wait for full recovery and not induce labor prematurely.

SAFETY/RISK ❖ **Supportive Treatments**

Most patients require supportive treatment only. Fetuses infected by Parvovirus B19 should be referred to tertiary care centers experienced in fetal cord blood sampling (cordocentesis) and fetal blood transfusion. A more aggressive approach favors cordocentesis for every fetus with evidence of fetal hydrops. Conservative physicians rely on the fact that the disease is self-limiting and resolves spontaneously in most cases and are wary of the potential adverse effects of invasive procedures.

Influenza Vaccination

Q I'm 27 years old and I recently learned that I'm pregnant. Now I realize that I must have been about 7 weeks pregnant when I took the influenza vaccine offered at work. Is my baby at risk of malformations?

A No evidence indicates that killed influenza vaccine is teratogenic, even if given during the first trimester. Since 1996, Health Canada's Centre for Disease Control and Prevention has recommended that pregnant women in their second and third trimesters be vaccinated. This should not be interpreted as evidence that the vaccine is teratogenic in the first trimester because such evidence does not exist.

In-Depth

Influenza is an acute respiratory illness brought on by virus types A or B. The disease causes rapid onset of fever, myalgia, malaise, sore throat, and nonproductive cough. The incubation period is 1 to 3 days, and the virus can undergo transition up to 7 days after the onset of illness. Complications, such as pneumonia, exacerbation of chronic illness, and even death, have been reported in North America during influenza epidemics.

Influenza vaccine consists of purified virus proteins. Because the virus changes its profile almost every year, researchers predict the form of influenza of the three most common strains of the virus, and the vaccine is prepared based on that. That is why annual immunization is needed.

SAFETY/RISK ❖ No Evidence

The risk of maternal and fetal illness and mortality from influenza seems to be greater than the theoretical risk of adverse effects on pregnancy outcome by the killed virus vaccine. There is no evidence that the vaccine is teratogenic, even if it is given during the first trimester.

The influenza vaccine is safe, effective, and cost-effective. It could prevent illness in 70% to 90% of healthy people younger than 65 years. The government of Ontario has recently decided to immunize all high-risk populations.

Adverse effects of the vaccine include a mild form of influenza and allergic reactions in people with allergy to eggs (the vaccine is manufactured using an egg substrate). Severe adverse effects are rare; Guillain-Barré Syndrome occurs in about 1 of every million people vaccinated.

FACT ✔ Vaccinate Against Influenza

Pregnant women face an increased risk of illness and stillbirth if they get influenza, as was shown in a few outbreaks in the 1910s and 1950s. Women with medical conditions that increase their risk of complications from influenza, such as chronic pulmonary or cardiac illness during the year before conception, should be vaccinated. In 1996, Health Canada's Centre for Disease Control and Prevention added pregnant women in their second and third trimesters to the list of high-risk populations they recommended be vaccinated. See www.cdc.gov/ncidod/diseases/flu/fluvac.htm.

Influenza Antigens

Because maternal influenza antigens can cross the placenta, vaccinating pregnant women could provide newborns with high antibody titers to the influenza virus that would protect them until self-immunization is likely to be protective. One study found that pregnant women responded to the vaccine the same way non-pregnant adults did. At delivery, almost half of 40 maternal-fetal pairs had notable antibody titer levels in neonatal cord serum. At 6 months old, only one infant had a detectable antibody level. The authors of this particular study recommended administration of a more potent influenza vaccine.

CMV Infection

Q I contracted a primary Cytomegalovirus (CMV) infection. What is the recommended waiting time between primary CMV infection and conception, and which tests are good for determining whether the infection period is over?

A Although no data on the proper waiting period between primary CMV infection and conception are available, we suggest waiting until CMV-specific immunoglobulin G (IgG) antibodies are present (at least 6 months). Intrauterine transmission of Cytomegalovirus (CMV) can occur whether a mother has prior immunity or acquires CMV for the first time during pregnancy. Most serious effects, however, have been noted only after primary maternal infection.

In-Depth

Cytomegalovirus is a common virus with worldwide distribution. It is transmitted horizontally (direct person-to-person contact with virus-containing secretions) and vertically (from mother to infant before, during, and after birth). It commonly causes infection during the perinatal period and during childhood. CMV ranges from the most common asymptomatic infections, especially in children, to enlargement of the liver and an infectious mononucleosis-like syndrome in mothers after the neonatal period.

FACT ✔ 1% of Live Births

Congenital CMV is seen in 1% of all live births in the United States. Intrauterine transmission from primary maternal infection occurs in 30% to 40% of cases, and approximately 5% to 25% of infected newborns experience intrauterine growth retardation, neonatal jaundice, purpura, microcephaly, brain damage, and other illnesses and effects. Acquired infections at birth or shortly thereafter from breast milk or cervical secretions are not associated with clinical neonatal illnesses.

Cytomegalovirus differs from other well-known causes of fetal infection, such as rubella and toxoplasmosis, because they produce congenital infection only if the mother acquires the infection immediately before or during pregnancy. In contrast, CMV can be transmitted from mother to fetus even when the mother is known to have been infected months or years before conception, as well as when primary infection occurs during pregnancy. Fortunately, congenital CMV infections in fetuses of women with immunity acquired before pregnancy are less likely to be clinically serious than those resulting from primary infection. Although the presence of antibodies in the mother before conception does not prevent transmission of CMV to her fetus, it helps prevent serious harm because it protects the newborn against symptoms and against later developments. The extent of this protection is not currently known.

SAFETY/RISK ❖ Latent Risk

To date, no data on the appropriate time CMV-infected women should wait before becoming pregnant are available. Available data lead us to suggest waiting until CMV-specific IgG antibodies are present (typically 6 months). Once a woman is infected with CMV, the virus can remain latent in her body for the rest of her life and can pass on to a fetus in any future pregnancy.

Antibodies

The amount of protection afforded a fetus by the antibodies its mother had before conception has been studied by comparing the outcomes of CMV-infected infants born to mothers who acquired primary CMV infection during pregnancy (primary-infection group) with those of CMV-infected infants born to mothers with immunity (recurrent-infection group). Only infants in the primary-infection group had symptomatic CMV infection at birth (18%); mental retardation, bilateral hearing loss, seizure, and death were seen only among children in this group. The chances of unilateral hearing loss (5% vs. 15%), chorioretinitis (2% vs. 6%), microcephaly (2% vs. 5%), and any CMV-related effects (8% vs. 25%) were lower in the recurrent-infection group. The authors concluded that the presence of maternal antibodies to CMV before conception provides substantial protection against damaging congenital CMV infection in newborns and that primary maternal infection during pregnancy is associated with more severe consequences to the baby.

Cancer Chemotherapy

Q My sister is 8-weeks pregnant and was diagnosed with stage 3 Hodgkin's disease last week. The oncologist suggests delaying chemotherapy until the second trimester. What are the effects of chemotherapy on a fetus after the first trimester? Where can I find reliable information on the subject?

A Available data suggest that exposure to chemotherapy during the first trimester of pregnancy is associated with increased risk of major malformations. Exposure during the second and third trimesters does not result in major malformations, but could have nonteratogenic effects, such as low birth weight. The brain develops throughout pregnancy, and it could be affected later in pregnancy.

In-Depth

Cancer occurs only rarely during pregnancy (incidence is 0.07% to 0.1%), but when it does it can put immense stress on the pregnant patient, her family, and physician. The current trend to defer pregnancy until later in life might lead to increased incidence of cancer during pregnancy. There is, however, very little information on the effect of pregnancy on cancer and the effects of cancer and its therapy on pregnancy outcome.

Although there are some controlled studies on the effects of chemotherapy on fetuses, most literature is based on either case reports or small, uncontrolled series. Most chemotherapeutic agents (cancer-fighting drugs) have been shown to damage rapidly dividing cells, such as bone marrow, intestinal epithelium, and reproductive organs. Animal studies suggest that a fetus would be similarly affected by these agents because fetal tissues have a high growth rate. This damage could result in spontaneous abortions or malformations.

FACT ✔ **Avoid Chemotherapy in First Trimester**

Chemotherapeutic drugs are potent teratogens. The risk of malformations when chemotherapy is administered during the first trimester has been estimated at 10% for single-agent chemotherapy and at 25% for combination chemotherapy. Thus, chemotherapeutic agents should be avoided during the first trimester.

There is no evidence of increased risk of teratogenesis during the second and third trimesters. A report on a small series of breast cancer patients confirmed that chemotherapy is effective and safe when administered after the first trimester. However, the long-term nonteratogenic effects of chemotherapy remain largely unknown. There have been reports of increased risk of stillbirth, low birth weight, and intrauterine growth retardation following treatment in the second and third trimesters. When chemotherapy is administered during pregnancy, delivery of the infant should be timed to avoid the worst chemotherapy adverse effects (i.e., on blood cells) and their associated problems.

The very limited available information does *not* suggest that children born to mothers treated with chemotherapy during pregnancy have impaired mental or physical development or that they will be infertile. Even less is known about the likelihood of second malignancies in these children. Antineoplastic agents administered systemically might reach clinically significant levels in breast milk, so breastfeeding is contraindicated.

RESOURCES

Consortium of Cancer in Pregnancy Evidence (CCoPE)

Clearly, there is still much to learn about the effects of cancer and cancer drugs during pregnancy and lactation. That is why Motherisk established the Consortium of Cancer in Pregnancy Evidence (CCoPE), an international group of oncologists, obstetricians, pediatricians, pharmacologists, geneticists, and specialists in related fields. CCoPE develops up-to-date, evidence-based information on diagnosis, management, prognosis, and effect on fetal outcome of cancer during pregnancy. Updated information is posted on the Cancer and Pregnancy section of the Motherisk website at www.motherisk.org/cancer.

Bacterial Vaginosis

Q *I'm pregnant and have just been diagnosed with bacterial vaginosis (BV) although I have no symptoms. Should I be treated?*

A There appears to be no benefit to screening or treating pregnant women with an average risk of BV. It is not even clear that treating pregnant women at high risk of BV is beneficial. However, if you and your doctor decide in favor of treatment, the drugs of choice are oral or intravaginal gel metronidazole or oral clindamycin. Both these drugs are safe to use throughout pregnancy.

In-Depth
Bacterial vaginosis (BV) occurs when there is an imbalance in vaginal bacteria. This relatively common condition affects between 9% and 23% of all pregnant women. It differs from other vaginal infections in its unique clinical signs and symptoms and the distinctive vaginal discharge associated with it.

Symptoms
Patients usually complain of itching and burning with a copious white discharge; vulvar or vaginal erythema (redness); or pain during intercourse and burning upon urination. Patients have a musty or fishy odor and a thin white vaginal discharge. Although it is generally believed to be an endogenous condition (arising from within the bacteria cell), some behavioral factors, such as use of contraceptives, use of intimate hygiene products, and smoking, are thought to be involved. Although it is not considered a true sexually transmitted infection, it does correlate with sexual activities. Almost half of all women diagnosed have neither signs nor symptoms.

Treatment Options
The United States Centers for Disease Control and Prevention recommend three different treatments for *non-pregnant women*: 500 mg of oral metronidazole twice daily for 7 days, one application of 2% clindamycin cream intravaginally at bedtime for 5 days, or one or two applications of intravaginal metronidazole gel for 5 days. One study showed that many women have tried over-the-counter remedies, such as acidophilus yogurt, vinegar douches, and boric acid. These preparations were not

only ineffective, but the women often misdiagnosed the vaginal infection and, therefore, instituted inappropriate treatment.

A report of five randomized controlled trials (RCTs) involving 1,504 women found that only women with a history of preterm birth appeared to benefit from treatment. Another RCT of 121 women found, however, that women treated for BV had a significantly lower rate of preterm births than untreated women did. Does this conflicting information mean all pregnant women should be routinely screened for BV? No clear answer can be found in the literature.

FACT ✔ **Adverse Outcomes**

A meta-analysis of 19 studies concluded that BV is an important risk factor for spontaneous abortions and premature births. Although BV can usually be eradicated, no clear evidence indicates that routine treatment of BV during pregnancy decreases adverse pregnancy outcomes. Most studies found that treatment did not reduce incidence of spontaneous abortions or premature labor.

Research Reviews

Several organizations, including the American Society of Obstetrics and Gynecology, the United States Preventive Services Task Force, the US Centers for Disease Control and Prevention, and the Canadian Task Force on Preventive Health Care, reviewed all the literature on this subject. They examined all RCTs of BV treatment that specifically measured pregnancy outcomes. Seven RCTs met the inclusion criteria for the meta-analysis. Results showed no benefit to treating women at average risk of BV. In fact, two trials of women with previous preterm deliveries indicated an increased risk of preterm delivery (less than 34 weeks gestation) in women who did not have BV but received treatment. The increased risk, however, could have been due to their history of preterm deliveries.

These researchers also found that the prevalence of BV has not been well studied; there were no population-based studies in the United States.

SAFETY/RISK ❖ **High-Risk Benefit**

There appears to be no benefit to screening and treating BV in the general population of pregnant women, but some pregnant women at high risk of BV might benefit from screening and treatment.

Untreated Depression

Q I'm currently taking an antidepressant for clinically diagnosed depression. Antidepressants have helped me greatly over the years. I've gotten to the point where I'm feeling well enough to start thinking about raising a family and would like to get pregnant. Does that mean that I must stop taking these drugs as soon as pregnancy is confirmed?

A The decision to continue or discontinue these drugs during pregnancy should be based on scientific evidence, not popular belief (often based on biased attitudes towards depression itself) about the use of psychotropic medications during pregnancy. Recent studies have documented the relative safety of these drugs, so you should not feel compelled to stop taking them when you become pregnant. What's more, not treating your depression during pregnancy carries risks of its own. If, however, after receiving appropriate evidence-based information, you decide to stop taking the drugs, you should be gradually tapered off them to avoid abrupt discontinuation syndrome.

In-Depth

Depression and anxiety disorders are common among women of childbearing age, and these women are often prescribed antidepressants. Although many of these drugs have been found not to be teratogenic, fear of taking them during pregnancy persists. For some reason, more fear appears to surround use of psychotropic drugs than surrounds other types of medication, probably because the illnesses for which they are prescribed even today still carry a certain stigma.

Hazardous Behaviors

Studies have found that mental illness can affect a mother's functional status and her ability to obtain prenatal care and avoid dangerous behavior. Mental illness can also affect decision-making capacities by causing cognitive distortions, and, because of this, it has been associated with poor attendance at antenatal clinics and malnutrition (which could lead to low birth-weight babies).

Depressed women are more likely to smoke and to use alcohol or other substances, which might compromise pregnancy. Depressed women can show deteriorating social function, emotional withdrawal, and excessive concern about their future ability to parent. They report excessive worry about pregnancy, are less likely to attend regular obstetric visits, and do not comply with prenatal advice. They take prenatal vitamins less often than non-depressed women and know less about the benefits of folic acid. These behaviors all predict poor pregnancy outcome.

Severe depression also carries the risk of self-injury, as well as psychotic, impulsive, and harmful behaviors that can affect pregnancy. When patients refuse treatment, physicians should monitor patients for crises, such as suicide attempts, deteriorating social function, psychosis, and inability to comply with obstetric advice.

> **FACT** ✔️
> **Physiologic Consequences**
> The literature examining risk of untreated depression during pregnancy suggests that psychopathologic symptoms during pregnancy have physiologic consequences for fetuses. It has also been postulated that depression results in hazardous behaviors that can indirectly affect obstetric outcomes.

Links to Adverse Outcomes

Untreated depression during pregnancy has been linked to other adverse outcomes, such as spontaneous abortion, increased uterine artery resistance, small head circumference, low Apgar scores, need for special neonatal care, neonatal growth retardation, preterm delivery, and babies with high cortisol levels at birth. Studies also suggest that pregnant women who are depressed require more operative deliveries and report labor as more painful, which means they require more epidural analgesia.

It is also evident that the risks of untreated depression do not end with birth. Women with untreated antenatal depression are also at increased risk of postpartum depression. Studies have shown that these women are less capable of carrying out maternal duties and of bonding with their children.

One study found elevated risk of preterm delivery (less than 37 weeks), low birth weight (less than 2500 g), and small

> **FACT** ✔️ **More Research Needed**
>
> Gestational hypertension and subsequent preeclampsia have also been linked to untreated depression during pregnancy. Psychopathology during pregnancy is thought to affect the uterine environment and, therefore, could have an effect on fetal outcome. Current theories suggest that depression increases excretion of vasoactive hormones in the mother, and these hormones then mediate birth outcome. More research is needed to find out the exact mechanism.

for gestational age (less than 10th percentile) babies in women with Beck Depression Inventory (BDI) scores of 21 or more who were not receiving treatment. Prenatal stress and depression have also been significantly associated with lower infant birth weight and younger gestational age at birth. A recent study of lower social class women found that depression was associated with restricted fetal growth and small for gestational age babies. There is also a clear association between increased hypothalamic, pituitary, and placental hormones in depressed mothers and the occurrence of preterm labor.

Studies have investigated the link between depression and preeclampsia. Strenuous work, depression, and anxiety might increase risk of this condition, but the stress of daily living has not been associated with it. In Finland, 623 nulliparous women (women who never bore children before) at low risk of preeclampsia all had healthy first trimesters and were then tested for depression and anxiety at about 12 weeks' gestation. Depression and anxiety were both associated with increased risk of preeclampsia.

Risk of Sudden Discontinuation

Antidepressants have an extremely low risk of abuse; they are not considered addictive agents. Symptoms of discontinuation can include general somatic, gastrointestinal, affective, and sleep disturbances that tend to occur abruptly within days to weeks of stopping or reducing the dose. Re-emergence of depression occurs more gradually. Reinstitution of antidepressants mitigates the symptoms of discontinuation within a day, but it might take several weeks for a beneficial effect on depression to be felt.

Motherisk recently published a study documenting the adverse effects of 36 women who called after abruptly discontinuing either antidepressants or benzodiazepines (28 had discontinued the medications on the advice of their physicians). Before becoming pregnant, these women had been functioning well with their depression well controlled. They stopped the medication only because they feared it would harm their babies. All the women suffered abrupt discontinuation syndrome;

FACT

Re-Emergence of Disorders

Another thing to beware of is sudden discontinuation of antidepressants, which can cause patients to experience discontinuation symptoms or re-emergence of the primary psychiatric disorder.

11 subsequently reported suicidal thoughts; and four were later hospitalized. One of the remaining women had a therapeutic abortion, and one substituted alcohol for a benzodiazepine. After Motherisk's counseling, two-thirds restarted their medication within several days. All babies born to mothers who restarted medication were normal and healthy.

SAFETY/RISK ❖ Evidence-Based Information

A growing body of literature suggests that the risk of adverse effects of untreated depression in pregnancy is high. When you compare that with the relative safety of antidepressants, the risk-benefit ratio seems clear. At the very least, be sure that your decision is based on all the available evidence-based information. Ask questions, get the answers, and make the best choice in consultation with your physician.

Guide to Safety/Risk of Medical Conditions in Pregnancy

The following table lists common medical conditions that may have to be treated and/or controlled during pregnancy. The information provided includes the effect of the condition on the course of pregnancy, as well as the effect of pregnancy on the condition. For example, rheumatoid arthritis tends to improve in pregnancy. In contrast, epileptic seizure may worsen for some women in late pregnancy.

This information does not cover every medical condition in pregnancy. If you can't find the information you need, please call a teratogen information service in your area, as listed in the "Resources" section of this book. A teratogen specialist is likely to know about the interactions between the condition and pregnancy. You may also want to consult a high-risk obstetrician or perinatologist.

MEDICAL CONDITION	EFFECT OF CONDITION ON PREGNANCY	EFFECT OF PREGNANCY ON CONDITION
AIDS/HIV	With optimal therapy: almost zero transmission. Without treatment: up to 50% transmission to baby.	Pregnancy does not affect the progress of AIDs.
Anemia	The most common medical complication in pregnancy. Can create risk for both mother and fetus. Appropriate iron supplementation is critical.	Significant maternal complications with hemoglobin lower than 60 g/L.
Antiphospholipid Antibodies: Lupus Anticoagulants and Anticardiolipin	Increased risk of recurrent miscarriage, fetal growth retardation, high risk of blood clots in mother.	Sometimes the condition becomes active only in pregnancy.
Asthma	Active asthma increases risk for prematurity, intrauterine growth retardation, perinatal mortality.	Severe asthma before pregnancy often predicts worsening during pregnancy. Attacks usually between weeks 28 to 36 of pregnancy. In 10% of cases, attacks start during labor. More frequent following cesarian section.
B-12 (vitamin) Deficiency	May be associated with infertility. Most fetuses are protected from such deficiency. When mother is B-12 deficient, breastfed infants may become deficient at 4 to 12 months.	Vitamin B-12 levels fall progressively in mother during pregnancy. Breastfeeding not recommended until the deficiency is corrected.
Cancer		
• Acute Leukemia	More spontaneous abortions, prematurity, stillbirth. Increased risk of maternal bleeding and infections. Cancer chemotherapy in first trimester associated with more congenital malformation.	Pregnancy does not affect course of cancer.

MEDICAL CONDITION	EFFECT OF CONDITION ON PREGNANCY	EFFECT OF PREGNANCY ON CONDITION
• Breast Cancer	Risk of malformations increase with chemotherapy in first trimester.	More metastatic disease in pregnancy.
• Cervical Cancer	Conization (removal of tumor) may increase risk of abortion, hemorrhage, rupture of membranes, prematurity.	Pregnancy does not affect survival.
• Hodgkin's Lymphoma	During first trimester, diagnostic or therapeutic radiation may risk the fetus.	Pregnancy does not affect survival.
• Melanoma	Sometimes, though rarely, maternal metastases are found in placenta or fetus.	Pregnancy does not affect survival.
• Ovarian Cancer	Increased risk of miscarriage, prematurity, fetal growth retardation.	Pregnancy does not affect survival.
Chlamydia Infection	In 50% of cases, may transmit to baby, causing eye infections, pneumonia. Other risks include premature rupture of membrane, prematurity, perinatal death, postpartum endometritis.	Pregnancy does not change the course of infection.
Cystic Fibrosis	In moderate to severe uncontrolled cases, may lead to maternal hypoxia and perinatal morbidity and mortality, prematurity, more gestational diabetes.	Increased risk for severe maternal disease and mortality in moderate to severe cases.
Cytomegalovirus (CMV) Infection	In most maternal infections: no maternal symptoms. In 40 to 80% of cases: the fetus will be infected. Congenital CMV: brain, eye, and hearing damage.	Pregnancy does not change the severity of maternal disease.

MEDICAL CONDITION	EFFECT OF CONDITION ON PREGNANCY	EFFECT OF PREGNANCY ON CONDITION
Depression	Untreated clinical depression can lead to relapse of symptoms. Depressed women have higher rates of obstetrical complications and preterm deliveries.	Tendency toward more depression in pregnancy and the risk of postpartum depression.
Diabetes Mellitus		
• **Type 1 Diabetes**	Increased rate of congenital malformation.	Increased insulin requirements. Pregnancy increases renal damage in women with diabetes nephropathy. Usually returns to pre-pregnancy value.
• **Type 2 Diabetes**	Large babies, increased perinatal mortality, birth trauma, respiratory distress syndrome, hypoglycemia.	Increased insulin requirements. Pregnancy increases renal damage in women with diabetes nephropathy. Usually returns to pre-pregnancy value.
• **Gestational Diabetes**	Large babies, increased perinatal mortality, birth trauma, respiratory distress syndrome, hypoglycemia, hypercalcemia.	Tends to arise in late pregnancy among women without previous diabetes.
Epilepsy	Epilepsy itself probably does not increase risk for congenital malformation. Increased risk for preeclampsia, prematurity, perinatal mortality.	Tendency toward more seizures in pregnancy.
Folic Acid Deficiency	Increased risk of neural tube defects (e.g., spina bifida).	Pregnancy aggravates folic acid depletion.

MEDICAL CONDITION	EFFECT OF CONDITION ON PREGNANCY	EFFECT OF PREGNANCY ON CONDITION
Gonorrhea Infection	The baby may be infected through ruptured membranes. Higher risk of premature rupture of membranes, prematurity chorioamvianitis. Baby's infection: eye, ear, throat, stomach, rectum, blood.	Pregnancy increases the risk of infection outside the cervix of uterus.
Heart Disease	Higher risk for miscarriage, fetal growth retardation. There is higher risk of congenital heart disease in the baby.	Cardiac output increases by 40% in late pregnancy — may deteriorate heart status. Pregnancy not recommended for high-risk cardiac lesions.
Hepatitis (viral)		
• **Hepatitis A**	No fetal infection with hepatitis A.	Pregnancy does not change the course of any of the hepatitis A, B, or C infections.
• **Hepatitis B**	Significant fetal infection with hepatitis B. More fetal mortality and prematurity.	Pregnancy does not change the course of any of the hepatitis A, B, or C infections.
• **Hepatitits C**	Significant fetal infection with hepatitis C. Only starts at third trimester.	Pregnancy does not change the course of any of the hepatitis A, B, or C infections.
• **Hepatitis E**	Disease increases fetal mortality and risk of prematurity.	May be more active and dangerous in pregnancy.
Herpes Simplex	Primary maternal infection may cause neonatal herpes: infection of brain, skin, or blood.	Primary maternal infections in pregnancy increase the risk of recurrence during labor.
Hypertension	Increased risk of preeclampsia. Increased risk of miscarriages, intrauterine growth retardation, placental abruption, prematurity, perinatal mortality.	Tendency to increase blood pressure and pregnancy — induced hypertension.

MEDICAL CONDITION	EFFECT OF CONDITION ON PREGNANCY	EFFECT OF PREGNANCY ON CONDITION
Hyperthyroidism	Risk of stillbirth, low birth weight, perinatal death, prematurity, preeclampsia.	Condition more common in first trimester and postpartum. No change in natural course of the condition.
Hypothyroidism	Decreased fertility. Tendency toward lower IQ in baby. If hypothyroidism is caused by iodine deficiency, then hypothyroidism and brain damage in baby is common.	In 20% of hypothyrotic women, more thyroid hormone is needed in pregnancy.
Immune Thrombocytopenia Purpura (ITP)	Increased risk of blood loss during delivery. Increased miscarriage. Increased fetal loss and fetal mortality.	ITP tends to worsen in pregnancy.
Inflammatory Bowel Disease (IBD)		
• **Crohn's Disease**	No clear evidence of adverse pregnancy outcome.	Pregnancy does not affect overall course. Majority enjoy remission. When Crohn's onset is in pregnancy, result may be severe course.
• **Ulcerative Colitis**	Increased miscarriage with ulcerative colitis.	Pregnancy does not affect overall course of condition.
Iron Deficiency Anemia	Higher risk for prematurity, intrauterine growth retardation, stillbirth, maternal death in developing countries.	Pregnancy itself is associated with lower hemoglobin and iron deficiency.
Malaria	Increased risk of fetal wastage. Intrauterine infection, placental insufficiency, intrauterine growth retardation, prematurity, low birth weight, stillbirth.	Pregnancy increases the severity of falciparum malaria.

MEDICAL CONDITION	EFFECT OF CONDITION ON PREGNANCY	EFFECT OF PREGNANCY ON CONDITION
Multiple Sclerosis	Flare-ups more common in first trimester and mainly after birth.	No effect of pregnancy on overall relapse rate. In severe disease: more infection, fatigue, and lung problems in pregnancy.
Parvovirus B19 (Fifth Disease)	Fetal infection in second half of pregnancy. Increased fetal loss, hemolytic anemia in fetus. Rarely, hydrops fetalis (cardiac failure secondary to anemia).	No effect of pregnancy on overall relapse rate. In severe disease, more infection, fatigue, and lung problems in pregnancy.
Renal (kidney) Disease	High risk of miscarriage prematurity. High risk of maternal anemia, preeclampsia, placental abruption.	Renal insufficiency may increase in pregnancy. High risk of hypertension.
Renal Transplant	Higher rates of miscarriage, premature rupture of membrane, prematurity.	Generally: glomerular filtration rate increases in normal pregnancy. Ideally: women should wait 2 balanced, healthy years after transplant before starting pregnancy.
Rheumatoid Arthritis	Small increased risk of fetal heart block if mother has AntiRo antibodies. Otherwise, no adverse effects on fetal outcome.	Tendency toward remission in pregnancy.
Rubella (German Measles)	Congenital rubella syndrome: eye lesions, deafness, heart effects, brain effects, intrauterine growth retardation. Highest risk in first trimester.	Pregnancy does not affect severity of condition.
Sickle Cell Disease	Higher risk of fetal wastage, miscarriage, infertility, prematurity, intrauterine growth retardation, perinatal death.	Chance of attacks increases in third trimester. Increased risk of heart failure, pyelonephritis, pulmonary embolism, and gallstones.

MEDICAL CONDITION	EFFECT OF CONDITION ON PREGNANCY	EFFECT OF PREGNANCY ON CONDITION
Streptococcus Group B	Preterm rupture of membranes, prematurity, severe infant infection with high mortality rate.	Usually no symptom in the pregnant woman.
Syphilis	Fetal infection in any trimester. Most severe fetal infection with first trimester exposure. Infant mortality, miscarriage, intrauterine growth retardation, stillbirth, abnormal skeletal development, eye problems, brain effects, fetal heart failure.	Pregnancy does not change the overall course of maternal syphilis.
Systemic Lupus Erythematosis	Increased stillbirths, intrauterine growth retardation, prematurity, perinatal mortality when disease is active. Increased risk of preeclampsia. Neonatal lupus syndrome: congenital heart block in minority of cases.	Pregnancy probably does not affect adversely the course of lupus.
Toxoplasmosis	Transmission to fetus at any time in pregnancy, but less likely in first trimester. High rates of adverse fetal effects: intrauterine growth retardation, jaundice, anemia, brain damage, hydrocephalus, mental retardation.	Pregnancy does not affect the course of disease.
Tuberculosis	Cases of fetal infection are rare.	No increased risk of progression to active disease in pregnancy.
Urinary Tract Infection	Intrauterine growth retardation, fetal death, prematurity.	More urinary tract infections in pregnancy.

MEDICAL CONDITION	EFFECT OF CONDITION ON PREGNANCY	EFFECT OF PREGNANCY ON CONDITION
Urolithioris (Renal Stone)	More risk of urinary tract infection.	Pregnancy does not affect course of condition. Increased stone passage in pregnancy. Fewer symptoms in pregnancy, and stones pass more easily.
Varicella (Chicken Pox)	Fetus may be infected, resulting in intrauterine growth retardation, limb damage, adverse brain development, mental retardation, eye damage. Risk mostly before 20 weeks of pregnancy.	Higher complication rate for infections in the mother during third trimester (e.g., risk of pneumonia).
Venous Thromboembolism	No fetal effects unless oral anticoagulants (coumadines) are given.	More clotting prevalence in pregnancy.

RESOURCES

Koren G, ed. Maternal-Fetal Toxicology. A Clinician's Guide. 3rd ed. New York: Marcel Dekker, 2001: Chapter 35.

CHAPTER TWELVE

Food, Nutritional Supplements, and Dieting

Q. *Now that I'm pregnant, do I have to eat more?*

— Motherisk Caller

A. *As your pregnancy progresses, you will want to gradually increase your daily energy intake.*

— Motherisk Counselor

Studies have shown that good nutrition has positive effects on the fetus, especially in terms of appropriate birth weight and decreased neonatal morbidity and mortality. Good nutrition also improves the recovery of the mother after giving birth.

Balanced Diet

Food Groups

You should carefully consider what you eat and consume foods from the basic food groups. The United States Department of Agriculture (USDA) Dietary Guidelines represented in the Food Guide Pyramid identify five food groups — the fats, oils, and sweets group; the milk, yogurt, and cheese group; the meat, fish, beans, eggs, and nut group; the vegetable group; the fruit group; and the bread, cereal, rice, and pasta group. Canada's Food Guide to Healthy Eating identifies four main food groups

— grain products; vegetables and fruit; milk products; and meat and alternatives. Both agencies recommend eating a balanced diet of these main food groups, with the USDA cautioning to use fats, oils, and sweets sparingly.

Pregnancy Needs

Pregnant and breastfeeding women need three to four servings of dairy products each day, around 300 calories more than before pregnancy, and 60 grams of protein a day. Foods with complex carbohydrates (such as rice, potatoes, and pasta) should make up at least 30% to 40% of the total calories per day.

Different women consume different amounts of calories every day, the average in North America being between 1900 to 2400 calories. During early pregnancy, women should increase their energy intake by 100 calories a day. In the second trimester, this should increase by 300 calories a day, and in the third trimester, 450 calories a day.

> **FACT** ✔
>
> **Low-Carb Diets**
> Low-carb diets
> in pregnancy and
> avoiding grains may
> deprive you of the
> benefit of folic acid
> supplementation
> of some foods.

Food Fears

Concerns have been raised about the fetal safety of certain foods eaten by mothers during pregnancy. Uncooked egg whites in desserts have been suspected of causing food poisoning that may affect the mother's health and, indirectly, the fetus, while listeria bacteria has been found in unpasteurized cheeses and uncooked delicatessen meats that may present a risk. The Environmental Protection Agency in the United States has warned against eating farmed salmon that may have dangerous levels of PCBs and dioxins, but the Food and Drug Administration has not issued a comparable caution. However, the FDA has advised pregnant women and nursing mothers to eat no more than 6 ounces of albacore tuna a week because of possible high mercury levels.

The list goes on ... and the advice is often confusing, if not downright contradictory. The fact is that there is insufficient evidence concerning the affects of the mother's food on the fetus to arrive at hard-and-fast conclusions. Much more work needs to be done in this field.

In the meantime, if you are concerned about any one food item, be sure to consult with your physician and a teratogen information center for reliable information and helpful advice. Do not make decisions based on rumors or guesses.

Food Guide Pyramid
A Guide to Daily Food Choices

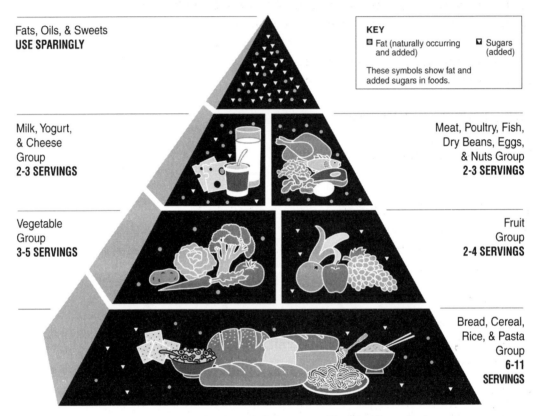

Fats, Oils, & Sweets
USE SPARINGLY

KEY
▫ Fat (naturally occurring and added)   ▾ Sugars (added)

These symbols show fat and added sugars in foods.

Milk, Yogurt, & Cheese Group
2-3 SERVINGS

Meat, Poultry, Fish, Dry Beans, Eggs, & Nuts Group
2-3 SERVINGS

Vegetable Group
3-5 SERVINGS

Fruit Group
2-4 SERVINGS

Bread, Cereal, Rice, & Pasta Group
6-11 SERVINGS

Source: U.S. Department of Agriculture/U.S. Department of Health and Human Services

The Food Guide Pyramid is an outline of what to eat each day based on the USDA Dietary Guidelines. It's not a rigid prescription but a general guide that lets you choose a healthful diet that's right for you.

The Pyramid calls for eating a variety of foods to get the nutrients you need and at the same time the right amount of calories to maintain healthy weight.

Use the Pyramid to help you eat better every day. Start with plenty of breads, cereals, rice, pasta, vegetables, and fruits. Add two to three servings from the milk group and two to three servings from the meat group. Remember to go easy on fats, oils, and sweets, the foods in the small tip of the Pyramid.

What Counts as One Serving?

The amount of food that counts as one serving is listed below. If you eat a larger portion, count it as more than one serving. For example, a dinner portion of spaghetti would count as two or three servings of pasta.

Be sure to eat at least the lowest number of servings from the five major food groups listed below. You need them for the vitamins, minerals, carbohydrates, and protein they provide. Just try to pick the lowest fat choices from the food groups. No specific serving size is given for the fats, oils, and sweets group because the message is USE SPARINGLY.

Milk, Yogurt, and Cheese
1 cup of milk or yogurt
$1\frac{1}{2}$ ounces of natural cheese
2 ounces of process cheese

Meat, Poultry, Fish, Dry Beans, Eggs, and Nuts
2-3 ounces of cooked lean meat, poultry, or fish
$\frac{1}{2}$ cup of cooked dry beans, 1 egg, or 2 tablespoons of
    peanut butter count as 1 ounce of lean meat

Vegetable
1 cup of raw leafy vegetables
$\frac{1}{2}$ cup of other vegetables, cooked or chopped raw
$\frac{3}{4}$ cup of vegetable juice

Fruit
1 medium apple, banana, orange
$\frac{1}{2}$ cup of chopped, cooked, or canned fruit
$\frac{3}{4}$ cup of fruit juice

Bread, Cereal, Rice, and Pasta
1 slice of bread
1 ounce of ready-to-eat cereal
$\frac{1}{2}$ cup of cooked cereal, rice, or pasta

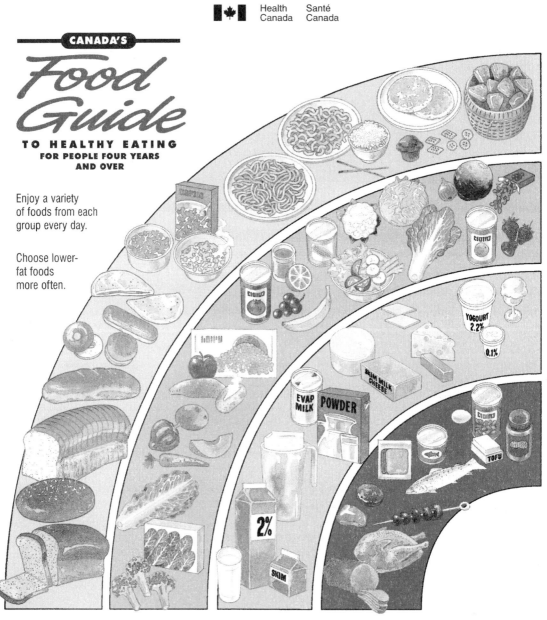

Health Canada   Santé Canada

CANADA'S
Food Guide
TO HEALTHY EATING
FOR PEOPLE FOUR YEARS AND OVER

Enjoy a variety of foods from each group every day.

Choose lower-fat foods more often.

Grain Products
Choose whole grain and enriched products more often.

Vegetables and Fruit
Choose dark green and orange vegetables and orange fruit more often.

Milk Products
Choose lower-fat milk products more often.

Meat and Alternatives
Choose leaner meats, poultry and fish, as well as dried peas, beans and lentils more often.

Canada

Grain Products

5 – 12

SERVINGS PER DAY

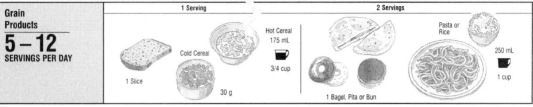

1 Serving — 1 Slice, Cold Cereal 30 g, Hot Cereal 175 mL 3/4 cup

2 Servings — 1 Bagel, Pita or Bun, Pasta or Rice 250 mL 1 cup

Vegetables and Fruit

5 – 10

SERVINGS PER DAY

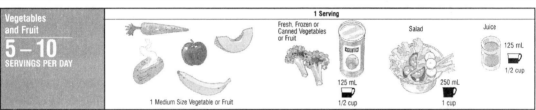

1 Serving — 1 Medium Size Vegetable or Fruit, Fresh, Frozen or Canned Vegetables or Fruit 125 mL 1/2 cup, Salad 250 mL 1 cup, Juice 125 mL 1/2 cup

Milk Products

SERVINGS PER DAY
Children 4–9 years: 2–3
Youth 10–16 years: 3–4
Adults: 2–4
Pregnant and Breast-feeding
Women 3–4

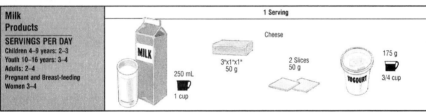

1 Serving — MILK 250 mL 1 cup, Cheese 3"x1"x1" 50 g, 2 Slices 50 g, Yogourt 175 g 3/4 cup

Other Foods

Taste and enjoyment can also come from other foods and beverages that are not part of the 4 food groups. Some of these foods are higher in fat or Calories, so use these foods in moderation.

Meat and Alternatives

2 – 3

SERVINGS PER DAY

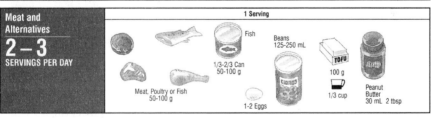

1 Serving — Meat, Poultry or Fish 50-100 g, Fish 1/3-2/3 Can 50-100 g, 1-2 Eggs, Beans 125-250 mL, Tofu 100 g 1/3 cup, Peanut Butter 30 mL 2 tbsp

Different People Need Different Amounts of Food

The amount of food you need every day from the 4 food groups and other foods depends on your age, body size, activity level, whether you are male or female and if you are pregnant or breast-feeding. That's why the Food Guide gives a lower and higher number of servings for each food group. For example, young children can choose the lower number of servings, while male teenagers can go to the higher number. Most other people can choose servings somewhere in between.

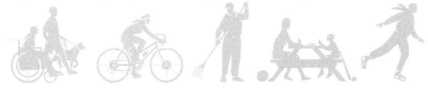

Consult *Canada's Physical Activity Guide to Healthy Active Living* to help you build physical activity into your daily life.

Enjoy eating well, being active and feeling good about yourself. That's VITALIT

© Minister of Public Works and Government Services Canada, 1997
Cat. No. H39-252/1992E   ISBN 0-662-19648-1

Vitamin and Mineral Supplements

Many women find it hard to supplement their diet with sufficient amounts of calcium, iron, and folic acid. Milk products, oranges, dark green vegetables and fruits, meat and/or legumes can help in meeting these needs, but you should also take a daily perinatal vitamin supplement that contains folic acid, iron, and calcium, along with other vitamins and minerals.

Pregnant women should not consume excessive doses of vitamins, though. Megadoses of vitamin A, for example, may increase the risk of brain and spinal malformations.

Weight Management

Different women experience different weight gain in pregnancy. Typically, weight gain of 6.8 to 18.2 kilograms (15 to 40 pounds) is considered optimal. This depends, of course, on pre-pregnancy weight. Underweight women are typically encouraged to achieve the higher range. It is not recommended that obese women lose weight during pregnancy.

Most people probably don't need to be reminded how hard it can be to lose weight once you've put it on. The same applies to excess weight gained in pregnancy. That's why it is important to eat properly and avoid overeating, particularly during mid to late pregnancy when an upsurge in corticosteroid hormones in the blood tends to cause an increase in appetite.

Dieting

Pregnancy is not the time to try high protein, low fat, low carb, crash, or fad diets. Acute, abrupt changes are not a safe approach in pregnancy.

Low-Carb Diets and Folic Acid

Q *It has been about a year-and-a-half since my last pregnancy and we've decided that we're ready to have a second child. Now I'm planning my next pregnancy. I gained a lot of weight in the first pregnancy, so I've been dieting for the past 6 months. I'm now on a low-carb diet and would like to know if it's okay to continue this diet once I get pregnant.*

A Your question couldn't be more timely! Your low-carb diet may be limiting your intake of folic acid, a micronutrient that is essential to the healthy development of the fetus. Quit the low-carb diet *now*, while you are planning. Don't wait until you are pregnant.

In-Depth

One of the most exciting breakthroughs in medical science was the discovery that folic acid, when consumed in sufficient amounts within the first weeks of pregnancy, could prevent neural tube defects (such as spina bifida) in the baby. Folic acid (a.k.a. folate and vitamin B-9) is found in leafy green vegetables (such as spinach), fruits (such as oranges), and legumes (such as lentils and kidney beans). The trouble is that not many women consume enough of these foods to get the 400 micrograms daily that are necessary to prevent neural tube defects. Attempts at educating women to consume folate before conception are not likely to succeed when 50% of pregnancies are unplanned.

FACT ✔ Folic Acid Fortification

In 1998, Health Canada called for the fortification of white flour and cornmeal with folic acid. In doing so, the Canadian government significantly improved the chance of preventing 400,000 affected births each year. The strategy seems to be working. The number of children born with neural tube defects is down by almost 50% and the incidence of neuroblastoma, a common childhood cancer, is down 60%.

Today, bread, pasta, breakfast cereals, and orange juice are valuable sources of folic acid. Those on low carb regimens, however, have eliminated these foods from their diets. While we do not suggest that you should rely entirely on bread and pasta for your folic acid intake (in fact, if white bread were your only source of folate, you would have to eat about eight slices daily to reach a minimum level), the better course is to maintain a healthy, balanced diet and take vitamin supplements containing folic acid throughout your reproductive years. If you have not been taking such vitamins, then start now, before conception. That way, you will be sure to have enough folic acid 'on board' in the first weeks of your pregnancy when your baby's neural tube is forming.

SAFETY/RISK ❖ Fad Diets

The benefits of folic acid and food supplementation are too important to sacrifice to fad diets. Nor is folic acid the only loss. Essential micronutrients, such as vitamin D and vitamin A, may also get lost in the mix.

Eating Fish

Q I am pregnant and feeling fine, but it seems every time you read the newspaper there's something new to worry about. I just read that tuna contains methylmercury, which is toxic to the fetal brain. I've been eating tuna throughout my pregnancy — just last week I had a couple of cans of tuna in one form or another. Is my baby at risk?

A Fresh tuna may contain toxic levels of methylmercury, but levels are much lower in canned tuna. Eating one or two cans of tuna (about 6 ounces) a week will not harm you or your baby.

In-Depth

Mercury is a toxin that attacks nerve cells. Inorganic mercury pollutes air, water, and soil through natural deposits, industrial and household disposal of wastes containing mercury, and use of fungicides that contain mercury.

When mercury is combined with carbon, organic mercury compounds are produced. The most common organic mercury is methylmercury (MeHg). Unlike inorganic mercury, organic mercury is readily absorbed through the gut. Methylmercury can contaminate seafood, and this raises concerns about whether it is safe for pregnant women to eat fish.

When there is mercury in the water, MeHg forms as a result of interaction with bacteria and subsequently builds up in the tissue of fish and other marine organisms. The most commonly used quantitative unit for measuring mercury concentration is parts per million (ppm), although micrograms per gram is sometimes used. Mercury intake is measured by microgram of mercury ingested per kilogram of body weight.

The nervous system is the main target of toxic doses of MeHg. Sensory, visual, and auditory function, and coordination are most commonly affected.

> **LOOK BACK**
>
> For more information on safe levels of mercury, see Chapter 10, "Chemical and Radiation Exposures."

Benefits and Risks of Seafood

Seafood is an important source of essential nutrients, including omega-3 polyunsaturated fatty acids and selenium. Essential fatty acids are necessary for optimal neurologic development, and they probably modify the effects of neurotoxins.

In Minamata, Japan, seafood heavily contaminated with MeHg caused an outbreak of congenital poisoning that resulted in a condition resembling spastic paresis (muscle tightness and weakness affecting the legs). In Iraq, an increase in the number of neurologic abnormalities was observed in infants whose mothers consumed mercury-poisoned grains and whose mothers' hair was found to have concentrations of mercury exceeding 10 ppm. Clinically, the extent of abnormalities in the fetus and infant depends on the level of exposure.

In 1971, a Swedish Expert Group conducted the first extensive evaluation of the health risks to humans of MeHg in fish. They concluded that the lowest level toxic to adults was 50 ppm (measured in the hair). A World Health Organization (WHO) expert group subsequently reaffirmed the Swedish conclusions and applied a safety factor of 10 to cover risk to the most sensitive subgroup of the population, which they assumed to be babies in the womb. Thus, 5 ppm was adopted as the international standard for the upper tolerable level of mercury (measured in mothers' hair).

FACT ✔ **Cerebral Palsy Symptoms**

Infants exposed to high levels of MeHg in their mothers' blood can present with cerebral palsy that is indistinguishable from the cerebral palsy caused by other factors. Microcephaly, impaired reflexes, and gross motor and mental impairment, sometimes associated with blindness or deafness, is the main pattern of abnormalities. Milder degrees of affliction are difficult to diagnose during the first few months of life, but they become obvious as time goes on. Patients mainly appear to have psychomotor difficulties and persistently impaired reflexes.

The WHO set guidelines for intake of mercury at 0.47 micrograms/kilogram of body weight daily. In 1996, the United States Environmental Protection Agency (EPA) set a new reference dose for MeHg at 0.1 microgram/kilogram of body weight daily, which was only one-fifth of the WHO dose. If the EPA's dose were followed, fish and seafood consumption would be drastically reduced.

Effects of MeHg on Two Island Populations

Some recent cohort studies have reported on MeHg consumption and developmental outcomes among children exposed to MeHg both before and after birth. One group of researchers studied children on one of the main Seychelles islands at $5\frac{1}{2}$ months old. Results of their study strongly supported findings in the same cohort at a younger age. These children had no neurodevelopmental deficits, even though their mothers' hair contained mean mercury concentrations of 6.8 ppm during pregnancy.

In the Faroe Islands, where MeHg exposure occurs primarily through consumption of pilot whale meat, analyses of 917 children at 7 years old found no clinical or neurophysiologic abnormalities related to mercury exposure. Subtle decreases in performance on neuropsychologic tests over time, however, were associated with prenatal levels of MeHg of less than 10 ppm in hair. Interestingly, the Faroese children had excellent visual contrast sensitivity that could be attributable to an ample supply of fish-borne omega-3 fatty acids.

Important differences between the two populations, such as nutritional practices, housing, and lifestyle, could explain the different outcomes, but the main difference was source of exposure. Ocean fish are the source of MeHg in the Seychelles, whereas pilot whales that contain a much higher level of MeHg (approximately 10 times higher) are the predominant source in the Faroe Islands. The latest study done on 182 newborns in the Faroe Islands shows that prenatal exposure to higher levels of MeHg from contaminated seafood is associated with higher risk of neurodevelopmental deficits.

SAFETY/RISK ❖ Government Guidelines

U.S.A. federal guidelines (1998) and Ontario Ministry of the Environment advice (1999) for pregnant women, women of childbearing age, and children under 15 both recommend:

- Eating only those fish designated with a clear fish symbol in the most recent guides for eating sport fish and consuming no more than four meals of such fish each month;
- Not eating any other categories of fish caught in freshwater lakes;
- Consuming no more than one meal of fresh shark, swordfish, or tuna each month;
- Not consuming sport fish if you are already a regular consumer of shark, swordfish, or fresh tuna; and
- Eating canned tuna because mercury levels in canned tuna are much lower than guideline levels.

RESOURCES

For more information, see Health Canada's " Nutrition for a Healthy Pregnancy — National Guidelines for the Childbearing Years." You can find it on-line at www.hc-sc.gc.ca.

CHAPTER THIRTEEN

Work, Exercise, and Sex during Pregnancy

Q. *I'm about 4 months pregnant and feeling fine. But people are telling me I may have to quit work and give up my weekly visits to the gym. Is this true?*

— *Motherisk Caller*

A. *So long as you are feeling fine and not experiencing any obstetric complications, you should be able to lead a fairly normal life. Depending on the work you do and the environment you work in, you may also find that you can continue to work throughout your pregnancy. Many women do. But you'll want to be sure that you are not exposing yourself or your baby to any harmful substances or engaging in what is defined below as 'strenuous work.' As for your weekly workout, discuss your regular routine with your doctor. Chances are, a mild weekly workout will do you well.*

— *Motherisk Counselor*

Strenuous Work

Today, many women need to continue working during pregnancy in order to help support their families. Many of these women are working outside the home. As a rule, for women with uncomplicated pregnancies, work does not appear to increase fetal risk. Women who work with chemicals need to know the risk nature of these chemicals because chemical solvents and heavy metals may affect the fetus. If you have a medical condition or have had a previous adverse obstetrical outcome, you should talk to your physician to see if your job is safe for you during pregnancy.

Physically challenging, strenuous work and more than 40-hour work weeks are associated with a small risk of prematurity and low birth weight.

WORKING TOO HARD

Strenuous work has been defined as:

- stooping and bending more than 10 times per hour

- repetitive climbing of ladders and poles (more than 3 times per 8-hour shift)

- repetitive lifting of more than 50 pounds (23 kg) after 20 weeks of gestation

- prolonged standing (more than 4 hours)

- lifting more than 24 pounds (11 kg) at 24 weeks of gestation

- repetitive stair climbing (more than 3 times per shift)

- intermittent stooping, bending, and ladder climbing after 28 weeks

- intermittent heavy lifting after 30 weeks or standing more than 30 minutes per hour after 32 weeks for healthy women

Exercise and Sports

Most women can exercise during pregnancy without risk to the fetus, but before you start, be sure to talk to your physician or other health-care provider.

Contraindications for Exercise

Conditions
- Previous obstetrical problems (e.g., incompetent cervix)
- Certain heart or lung problems
- Certain uncontrolled metabolic conditions (e.g., type 1 diabetes mellitus, or thyroid disease)
- Infectious diseases (e.g., infectious mononucleosis, hepatitis)
- Multiple pregnancy
- Poor nutrition
- Low maternal fat stores
- Use of certain medications

Positions
The supine position should be avoided and abdominal exercise should be performed in the side-lying or standing position.

Rough Sports
Sports that involve potential injury, falls, or blows should be avoided or modified, including downhill skiing and mountain climbing. Scuba diving and water skiing should be avoided during pregnancy.

RECOMMENDED EXERCISES AND PRECAUTIONS

Exercises Encouraged in Pregnancy
- Walking
- Swimming
- Stationary Cycling
- Low-impact Aerobics

Precautions during Pregnancy
Before your exercise, be sure to do 10 to 15 minutes of warm-up and stretches. Also be sure you have adequate breast support. Workouts should typically be 15 to 30 minutes long, with appropriate breaks and fluid intake. A gradual 10- to 15-minute cooldown will prevent effects on the fetal heart rate. Women who exercise may also need higher caloric intake than the recommended amounts outlined in our discussion on nutrition during pregnancy.

MODIFIED HEART RATE TARGET ZONES FOR AEROBIC EXERCISE IN PREGNANCY

The level of exercise depends on your general fitness and your level of exercise before pregnancy. The intensity of the exercise is typically measured by maximal heart rate. The following Modified Heart Rate Target Zones for Aerobic Exercise in Pregnancy are based on age and apply to healthy women:

Age	Heart Rate Target Zone (beats/min)
Less than 20	140 – 155
20 - 29	135 – 150
30 - 39	130 – 145
40 or older	125 – 140

Sauna and Jacuzzi

An increase in core body temperature is associated with an increased risk of neural tube defects in the fetus. That's why you should not exercise in an exceedingly warm or humid environment, or use saunas or jacuzzis for extended periods of time.

Sexual Intercourse

If you are healthy, you can enjoy your sexuality and sexual relations throughout pregnancy without risk to you or to your unborn baby. When there is a risk of threatened abortion, antepartum hemorrhage, or threatened preterm labor, your physician should discuss with you the appropriate extent of sexual activity, various safe positions, and pleasuring techniques.

RESOURCES

Workplace Reproductive Health, Research and Strategies. Best Start: Ontario's Maternal Newborn and Early Child Development Resource Centre, 2001.

Visit the Occupational and Environmental Exposures page of the Motherisk website at www.motherisk.org/enviro/index.php.

CHAPTER FOURTEEN
Breastfeeding and Drugs

Q. How much of my medication will reach my nursing baby?

— *Motherisk Caller*

A. Most medications are excreted into breast milk in very small quantities. This means that typically, your baby will receive very small amounts of the drug, even after we consider the difference between your body weight and that of your child.

— *Motherisk Counselor*

Breast milk is the best food for the newborn and infant, largely because it contains nutrients and antibodies that help fight infection. However, if you are taking medication, your decision to breastfeed your baby and/or continue your medication will depend on several important considerations.

Some women decide not to breastfeed so they won't transfer their medications to the baby through their breast milk. Other women choose to breastfeed but discontinue their medications. Though these 'all or nothing' approaches are aimed at protecting the nursing child, they may not be the best choice for mother and baby. We suggest that a third, more rational and medically sound approach is to determine how much medication will reach your baby through the breast milk and whether that amount is known to be harmful.

5% Guideline

An unofficial guideline is that when the baby is exposed to less than 5% of the drug that the breastfeeding mother is exposed to per kilogram of body weight, it is very unlikely that the baby will suffer adverse effects. Very few medications result in baby's exposure at greater than 5%. Very simply, the vast majority of medicinal drugs are compatible with breastfeeding. This is what the American Academy of Pediatrics believes, as does the Motherisk Program.

Nevertheless, there are certain medications, even at this low level of transfer from mother to child, that are not safe.

For other drugs, which may be excreted at higher levels into milk, continuation of breastfeeding must be done in conjunction with appropriate expert monitoring, including measurement of the drug in the breast milk and sometimes also in the baby.

It is also important to follow the baby carefully for any unusual symptom. For example, if you need a drug for sleeplessness (such as the Valium derivative, clonazepam), and upon starting it, your baby appears to be more sleepy, it may mean that your child is sensitive even to the small amounts of the drug that reach the breast milk. In this example, a physician may need to prescribe another medication or may recommend that you discontinue breastfeeding. This sort of assessment should be done by the physician caring for the baby.

GUIDE TO MEDICATIONS AND AGENTS THAT MAY NOT BE SAFE FOR NURSING INFANTS

Drug	Risk to Infant
Amiodarone	Large exposure by suckling baby. High content of iodine. Levels in the milk can be individually measured to estimate accurately the child's exposure.
Lithium	Large exposure by some babies. Levels in milk and baby can assist in defining if there is a risk.
Phenobarbital	Large exposure by suckling baby. May cause sleepiness and chemical dependence.
Radioactive Agents	May expose the baby for risks of radiation. Includes radionuclides such as radioactive iodine used for diagnostic imaging.
Tetracycline	May adversely affect tooth development.

Guide to Selected Medications Compatible with Breastfeeding

GENERIC MEDICATION	RECOMMENDED FOLLOW-UP FOR CHILD
PAIN RELIEVERS	
Acetaminophen	Nothing specific. Talk to your pediatrician if unusual symptoms occur.
Codeine, Meperidine, Morphine	Follow for sleepiness, constipation.
ANTIBIOTICS	
Amoxicillin, Ampicillin, Cephalexin, Cefadroxil, Ciprofloxacin, Clindamycin, Cloxacillin, Erythromycin, Nalidixic Acid, Ofloxacin, Penicillin, Sulfamethoxazole, Trimethoprim, Vancomycin	Antibiotics in this group may affect the growth of bacteria in baby's gut. Follow-up for diarrhea.
ANTI-INFECTIVES	
Acyclovir, Chloroquine, Hydroxychloroquine, Isoniazid, Ketoconazole, Metronidazole	None needed.
ANTIEPILEPTICS	
Carbamazepine, Phenytoin, Valproic Acid	Follow-up for sleepiness in this group.
ANTIDEPRESSANTS	
Amitryptiline, Clomipramine, Desipramine, Doxepin, Fluoxetine, Fluvoxamine, Imipramine, Nortryptiline, Paroxetine, Sertraline, Trazodone, Zopiclone	Follow-up for potential discontinuation syndrome in this group.
ANTIHISTAMINES	
Loratadine, Tripolidine	Nothing specific. Talk to your pediatrician if unusual symptoms occur.
Old Antihistamines	Follow-up for sedation.
ANTIHYPERTENSIVES	
Atenolol, Captopril, Clonidine, Diltiazem, Enalapril, Hydralazine, Labetolol, Methyldopa, Metoprolol, Nadolol, Nifedipine, Nitrendipine, Propranolol, Sotalol, Timolol	Low blood pressure in baby may cause baby to look sick. Follow-up for adverse reactions in this group.

GENERIC MEDICATION	RECOMMENDED FOLLOW-UP FOR CHILD
ANTI-INFLAMMATORIES	
Aspirin, Diclofenac, Ibuprofen, Indomethacin, Ketorolac, Naproxen, Piroxicam, Prednisolone	Nothing specific. Talk to your pediatrician if unusual symptoms occur.
ANTIPSYCHOTICS	
Chlorpromazine, Haloperidol, Perphenazine, Risperidone, Zyprexa	Follow-up for sleepiness in this group.
ANTITHYROIDS	
Methimazole, Propylthiouracil	Follow thyroid function in the baby.
SEDATIVE ANXIOLYTICS	
Alprazolam, Clonazepam, Diazepam, Lorazepam, Midazolam, Nitrazepam, Oxazepam, Temazepam	Follow-up for sleepiness and withdrawal in this group.
CARDIOVASCULAR DRUGS	
Digoxin, Disopyramide, Flecainide, Mexiletine, Procainamide, Propafenone, Quinidine	Nothing specific. Talk to your pediatrician if unusual symptoms occur.
DIURETICS	
Acetazolamide, Chlorothiazide, Furosemide, Hydrochlorothiazide, Spironolactone	Follow-up for urine production and dehydration in this group.
GASTROINTESTINAL DRUGS	
5-Aminosalicylic, Cisapride, Famotidine, Loperamide, Metoclopramide, Ranitidine	Follow baby for any unusual symptoms, especially with regard to bowel movements and vomiting.
MISCELLANEOUS	
Pseudoephedrine	Follow baby for irritability.
Sumatriptan	Nothing specific. Talk to your pediatrician if unusual symptoms occur.
Warfarin	Follow baby for bleeding (though this is very unlikely to occur).

Drinking Alcohol while Breastfeeding

Q *I recently delivered a healthy, full-term baby and am now breastfeeding exclusively. I abstained from drinking alcohol during my entire pregnancy and am wondering if drinking alcohol now would harm my nursing baby.*

A Nursing mothers who choose to drink alcohol during the postpartum period should carefully plan a breastfeeding schedule by storing milk before drinking and waiting for complete elimination of alcohol from their breast milk after drinking. Motherisk has created an algorithm to estimate how long it takes to eliminate alcohol from breast milk.

In-Depth

While ample evidence indicates that drinking alcohol during pregnancy poses a severe and avoidable risk to the fetus, the risks of drinking alcohol while breastfeeding are not well defined. Currently, some mothers are still advised by physicians, nurses, lactation consultants, family members, and friends that it is all right to drink, even though a safe level of alcohol in breast milk has never been established.

Alcohol consumed by a mother passes easily into her breast-milk at concentrations similar to those found in her bloodstream. A nursing infant is actually exposed to only a fraction of the alcohol the mother ingests, but infants detoxify alcohol in their first weeks of life at only half the rate of adults.

FACT ✔ **Potential Adverse Effects**

Several proven or potential adverse effects of alcohol on nursing infants have been reported, even after exposure to only moderate levels: impaired motor development, changes in sleep patterns, decrease in milk intake, and risk of hypoglycemia. In addition, drinking large amounts of alcohol could affect lactating women's milk flow.

Some report that beer aids milk production and that infants prefer alcohol-flavored breast milk. Even though beer may increase maternal milk production and alcohol affects its flavor, evidence indicates that the presence of alcohol in breast-milk has an overall effect of decreasing infant consumption by 23%. The underlying mechanism for this reduction is unknown.

Occasional drinking while nursing has not been associated with overt harm to the infant. And since breast milk is such an important source of nutrients and immunities for the baby, occasional drinking while nursing should not be taken as a reason to stop breastfeeding. The possibility of adverse effects has not been ruled out, nor are there any known benefits of exposing nursing infants to alcohol.

SAFETY/RISK ❖ Avoid Exposure

Until a safe level of alcohol in breast milk is established, the safest choice is to avoid exposure to the nursing infant. Carefully planning a breastfeeding schedule and waiting for complete alcohol clearance from breast milk can help you do that.

ALCOHOL CLEARANCE FROM BREAST MILK CALCULATION

The Motherisk team has developed a formula to help breastfeeding mothers and their health-care providers determine how long it takes to eliminate alcohol completely from breast milk. It represents the time from beginning of drinking until the alcohol's clearance from breast milk for women of various body weights and average height (5'4") and assumes that alcohol metabolism is constant at 15 mg/dL. For example, if a woman weighs 90 pounds and consumes three drinks in 1 hour, it will take 8 hours, 30 minutes for there to be no alcohol in her breast milk. For a 210-pound woman drinking the same amount, it will take 5 hours, 33 minutes. Similarly, if a 140-pound woman drinks four bottles of beer starting at 8:00 p.m., it will take 9 hours, 17 minutes for there to be no alcohol in her breast milk (i.e., until 5:17 a.m.).

Note:

Drinking water, resting, or 'pumping and dumping' breast milk will not accelerate elimination. Unlike urine, which stores substances in the bladder, alcohol is not trapped in breast milk, but is constantly removed as it diffuses back into the bloodstream.

Mother's Weight kg (lbs)	No. of Drinks (Hours : Minutes) 1 drink = 340 g (12 oz) of 5% beer, or 141.75 g (5 oz) of 11% wine, or 42.53 g (1.5 oz) of 40% liquor.											
	1	**2**	**3**	**4**	**5**	**6**	**7**	**8**	**9**	**10**	**11**	**12**
40.8 (90)	2:50	5:40	8:30	11:20	14:10	17:00	19:51	22:41				
43.1 (95)	2:46	5:32	8:19	11:05	13:52	16:38	19:25	22:11				
45.4 (100)	2:42	5:25	8:08	10:51	13:34	16:17	19:00	21:43				
47.6 (105)	2:39	5:19	7:58	10:38	13:18	15:57	18:37	21:16	23:56			
49.9 (110)	2:36	5:12	7:49	10:25	13:01	15:38	18:14	20:50	23:27			
52.2 (115)	2:33	5:06	7:39	10:12	12:46	15:19	17:52	20:25	22:59			
54.4 (120)	2:30	5:00	7:30	10:00	12:31	15:01	17:31	20:01	22:32			
56.7 (125)	2:27	4:54	7:22	9:49	12:16	14:44	17:11	19:38	22:06			
59.0 (130)	2:24	4:49	7:13	9:38	12:03	14:27	16:52	19:16	21:41			
61.2 (135)	2:21	4:43	7:05	9:27	11:49	14:11	16:33	18:55	21:17	23:39		
63.5 (140)	2:19	4:38	6:58	9:17	11:37	13:56	16:15	18:35	20:54	23:14		
65.8 (145)	2:16	4:33	6:50	9:07	11:24	13:41	15:58	18:15	20:32	22:49		
68.0 (150)	2:14	4:29	6:43	8:58	11:12	13:27	15:41	17:56	20:10	22:25		
70.3 (155)	2:12	4:24	6:36	8:48	11:01	13:13	15:25	17:37	19:49	22:02		
72.6 (160)	2:10	4:20	6:30	8:40	10:50	13:00	15:10	17:20	19:30	21:40	23:50	
74.8 (165)	2:07	4:15	6:23	8:31	10:39	12:47	14:54	17:02	19:10	21:18	23:50	
77.1 (170)	2:05	4:11	6:17	8:23	10:28	12:34	14:40	16:46	18:51	20:57	23:03	
79.3 (175)	2:03	4:07	6:11	8:14	10:18	12:22	14:26	16:29	18:33	20:37	22:40	
81.6 (180)	2:01	4:03	6:05	8:07	10:08	12:10	14:12	16:14	18:15	20:17	22:19	
83.9 (185)	1:59	3:59	5:59	7:59	9:59	11:59	13:59	15:59	17:58	19:58	21:58	23:58
86.2 (190)	1:58	3:56	5:54	7:52	9:50	11:48	13:46	15:44	17:42	19:40	21:38	23:36
88.5 (195)	1:56	3:52	5:48	7:44	9:41	11:37	13:33	15:29	17:26	19:22	21:18	23:14
90.7 (200)	1:54	3:49	5:43	7:38	9:32	11:27	13:21	15:16	17:10	19:05	20:59	22:54
93.0 (205)	1:52	3:45	5:38	7:31	9:24	11:17	13:09	15:02	16:55	18:48	20:41	22:34
95.3 (210)	1:51	3:42	5:33	7:24	9:16	11:07	12:58	14:49	16:41	18:32	20:23	22:14

CHAPTER FIFTEEN

Resources

Teratogen Information Centers and Resources

Motherisk

The Motherisk Program at The Hospital for Sick Children in Toronto, Canada is one of the biggest teratogen research, counseling, and education centers in the world. It is the only such program in Canada. You can learn more about Motherisk by visiting www.motherisk.org.

European Network Teratogen Information Services (ENTIS)

The European Network Teratogen Information Services (ENTIS) represents member services throughout Europe, Israel, and parts of South America. If you are looking for teratogen information services abroad, try reviewing the list of ENTIS members at www.entis-org.com.

Organization of Teratology Information Services (OTIS)

The Organization of Teratogen Information Services (OTIS) represents member services in North America. For information regarding OTIS or the Teratology Information Service in your area, contact OTIS Information at: (866) 626-OTIS or (866) 626-6847. Information about OTIS is also available on-line at www.otispregnancy.org/index.htm.

OTIS members also provide telephone counseling to the public in various states and provinces in North America:

Alabama
Alabama Birth Defects Surveillance
University South Alabama
Department Medical Genetics
307 University Boulevard, Rm. 214, CC/CB
Mobile, AL 36688-0002
Tel. (800) 423-8324 or (334) 460-7691

Arizona
Arizona Teratogen Information Program
University of Arizona
PO Box 245079
Tucson, AZ 85724-5079
Tel. (888) 285-3410 or (520) 626-3410

California
CTIS Pregnancy Risk Information
UCSD Medical Center, Department of Pediatrics
200 W. Arbor Drive, #8446
San Diego, CA 92103-8446
(800) 532-3749 (California only)

Illinois
Illinois Teratogen Information Service
680 N. Lake Shore Drive, Suite 1230
Chicago, IL 60611
Tel. (800) 252-4847 (IL only) or (312) 981-4354

Indiana, Kentucky, Ohio
Indiana Teratogen Information Service
Indiana University Medical Center
Department of Medical and Molecular Genetics 1B130
975 W. Walnut Street
Indianapolis, IN 46202-5251
Tel. (317) 274-1071

Massachusetts, Maine, New Hampshire, Rhode Island
Massachusetts Teratogen Information Service (MaTIS)
Pregnancy Environmental Hotline
40 Second Avenue, Suite 520
Waltham, MA 02451
Tel. (800) 322-5014 (MA only) or (781) 466-8474

Missouri

Missouri Teratogen Information Service
University of Missouri Hospital and Clinics
One Hospital Drive, DC 05800
Columbia, MO 65212
Tel. (800) 645-6164 or (573) 884-1345

Nebraska

Nebraska Teratogen Project
University of Nebraska Medical Center
985440 Nebraska Medical Center
Omaha, NE 68198-5440
Tel. (402) 559-5071

New Jersey, Delaware, Pennsylvania

Pregnancy Healthline
Southern New Jersey Perinatal Cooperative
2500 McClellan Avenue, Suite 110
Pennsauken, NJ 08109-4613
Tel. (888) 722-2903 (NJ only) or (856) 665-6000

New York

Pregnancy Risk Network
976 Delaware Avenue
Buffalo, NY 14209
Tel. (800) 724-2454 (then press 1) (NY only)
or (716) 882-6791 (then press 1)

PEDECS
University of Rochester Medical Center
Department of Obstetrics and Gynecology
601 Elmwood Avenue
Rochester, NY 14642-8668
Tel. (716) 275-3638

North Carolina

Fetal Alcohol and Drug Program
Department of Pediatrics / Medical Genetics
Wake Forest University School of Medicine
Medical Center Boulevard
Winston-Salem, NC 27157-1076
Tel. (800) 532-6302

Ontario
Motherisk Program
The Hospital For Sick Children
555 University Avenue
Toronto, ON M5G 1X8
Main Call Center (416) 813-6780
Alcohol and Substance Use Helpline (877) 327-4636
Nausea and Vomiting of Pregnancy Helpline (800) 436-8477
HIV and HIV Treatment in Pregnancy (888) 246-5840

Quebec
IMAGE: Info-Medicaments en Allaitement et Grossesse
Pharmacy Dept. Ste. Justine Hospital
Montreal, QC H3T 1C5
Tel. (514) 345-2333

Texas
Texas Teratogen Information Service
UNT Department of Biology
PO Box 305220
Denton, TX 76203-5220
Tel. (800) 733-4727 or (940) 565-3892

Utah, Montana
Pregnancy RiskLine
Utah Department of Health
PO Box 144691
Salt Lake City, UT 84114-4691
Tel. (801) 328-2229 or (800) 822-2229

Washington, Alaska, Idaho, Oregon
CARE Northwest
University of Washington
PO Box 357920
Seattle, WA 98195-7920
Tel. (888) 616-8484

West Virginia
West Virginia University Hospitals
Physician Office Center
PO Box 782
OBGYN Clinic
Morgantown, WV 26507
Tel. (304) 293-1572

Wisconsin

Wisconsin Teratogen Information Service
347 Waisman Center
1500 Highland
Madison, WI 53705
Tel. (800) 442-6692

Workplace Hazards to Reproductive Health
Bureau of Occupational Health, Rm. B157
PO Box 2659
Madison, WI 53702-2659
Tel. (608) 266-2074
Fax. (608) 266-1550

Index

Z